Neurorhinology: Common Pathologies

Guest Editors

RICHARD J. HARVEY, MD
CARL H. SNYDERMAN, MD

OTOLARYNGOLOGIC CLINICS OF NORTH AMERICA

www.oto.theclinics.com

August 2011 • Volume 44 • Number 4

SAUNDERS an imprint of ELSEVIER, Inc.

W.B. SAUNDERS COMPANY

A Division of Elsevier Inc.

1600 John F. Kennedy Boulevard ● Suite 1800 ● Philadelphia, Pennsylvania 19103-2899

http://www.theclinics.com

OTOLARYNGOLOGIC CLINICS OF NORTH AMERICA Volume 44, Number 4
August 2011 ISSN 0030-6665, ISBN-13: 978-1-4557-1116-1

Editor: Joanne Husovski
Developmental Editor: Donald Mumford

Otolaryngologic Clinics of North America (ISSN 0030-6665) is published bimonthly by Elsevier, Inc., 360 Park Avenue South, New York, NY 10010-1710. Months of issue are February, April, June, August, October, and December. Business and Editorial Offices: 1600 John F. Kennedy Blvd., Suite 1800, Philadelphia, PA 19103-2899. Customer Service Office: 6277 Sea Harbor Drive, Orlando, FL 32887-4800. Periodicals postage paid at New York, NY and additional mailing offices. Subscription prices is $310.00 per year (US individuals), $590.00 per year (US institutions), $149.00 per year (US student/resident), $409.00 per year (Canadian individuals), $741.00 per year (Canadian institutions), $459.00 per year (international individuals), $741.00 per year (international institutions), $230.00 per year (international & Canadian student/resident). Foreign air speed delivery is included in all *Clinics'* subscription prices. All prices are subject to change without notice. **POSTMASTER:** Send address changes to *Otolaryngologic Clinics of North America*, Elsevier Health Sciences Division, Subscription Customer Service, 3251 Riverport Lane, Maryland Heights, MO 63043. **Telephone: 1-800-654-2452 (U.S. and Canada); 314-447-8871 (outside U.S. and Canada). Fax: 314-447-8029. E-mail: journalscustomerservice-usa@elsevier.com (for print support); journalsonlinesupport-usa@elsevier.com (for online support).**

Reprints. For copies of 100 or more of articles in this publication, please contact the Commercial Reprints Department, Elsevier Inc., 360 Park Avenue South, New York, NY 10010-1710. Tel.: 212-633-3812; Fax: 212-462-1935; E-mail: reprints@elsevier.com.

Otolaryngologic Clinics of North America is also published in Spanish by McGraw-Hill Interamericana Editores S.A., P.O. Box 5-237, 06500 Mexico D.F., Mexico.

Otolaryngologic Clinics of North America is covered in *MEDLINE/PubMed (Index Medicus), Current Contents/Clinical Medicine, Excerpta Medica, BIOSIS, Science Citation Index,* and *ISI/BIOMED.*

Printed and bound by CPI Group (UK) Ltd, Croydon, CR0 4YY

Transferred to Digital Print 2011

Contributors

GUEST EDITORS

RICHARD J. HARVEY, MD
Associate Professor, University of New South Wales/Macquarie University, Department of Otolaryngology/Skull Base Surgery, St Vincent's Hospital, Sydney, Australia

CARL H. SNYDERMAN, MD, MBA
Professor, Departments of Otolaryngology and Neurological Surgery, University of Pittsburgh School of Medicine; Co-Director, Center for Cranial Base Surgery, University of Pittsburgh Medical Center, Pittsburgh, Pennsylvania

AUTHORS

NITHIN D. ADAPPA, MD
Assistant Professor, Department of Otorhinolaryngology–Head and Neck Surgery, University of Pennsylvania School of Medicine, Hospital of the University of Pennsylvania, Philadelphia, Pennsylvania

MORAN AMIT, MD
Department of Otolaryngology–Head and Neck Surgery, Tel Aviv Sourasky Medical Center, Tel Aviv University, Tel Aviv, Israel

BENG TI ANG, MBBS, FRCSEd(SN)
Professor of Neurosurgery, Department of Neurosurgery, National Neuroscience Institute, Singapore

LEONARDO BALSALOBRE, MD
São Paulo ENT Center, Professor Edmundo Vasconcelos Hospital; Department of Otolaryngology–Head and Neck Surgery, Federal University of São Paulo, São Paulo, Brazil

ANGELA BLOUNT, MD
Fourth Year Resident, Division of Otolaryngology–Head and Neck Surgery, University of Alabama at Birmingham, Birmingham, Alabama

ALEXANDER G. CHIU, MD
Division Chief, Division of Otolaryngology–Head and Neck Surgery, Arizona Health Science Center, University of Arizona, Tucson, Arizona

RATAPHOL CHRIS DHEPNORRARAT, MBBS, FRACS
Rhinology Fellow, Department of Otorhinolaryngology, Singapore General Hospital, Singapore

JUAN FERNANDEZ-MIRANDA, MD
Assistant Professor, Department of Neurological Surgery, University of Pittsburgh School of Medicine, Pittsburgh, Pennsylvania

DAN M. FLISS, MD
Department of Otolaryngology–Head and Neck Surgery, Tel Aviv Sourasky Medical Center, Tel Aviv University, Tel Aviv, Israel

WYTSKE J. FOKKENS, MD, PhD
Department of Otolaryngology, Academic Medical Centre, Amsterdam, The Netherlands

PAUL A. GARDNER, MD
Assistant Professor, Department of Neurological Surgery, University of Pittsburgh School of Medicine; Co-Director, Center for Cranial Base Surgery, University of Pittsburgh Medical Center, Pittsburgh, Pennsylvania

CHRISTOS GEORGALAS, PhD, DLO, FRCS(ORL-HNS)
Department of Otolaryngology, Co-Director, Endoscopic Skull Base Centre, Academic Medical Centre, Amsterdam, The Netherlands

ZIV GIL, MD, PhD
Head and Neck Surgery Unit, Department of Otolaryngology–Head and Neck Surgery, Tel Aviv Sourasky Medical Center, Tel Aviv University, Tel Aviv, Israel

JOHN GOUDAKOS, MD
Department of Otolaryngology, AHEPA University Hospital, Aristotle University of Thessaloniki, Thessaloniki, Greece

JERRY R. GREENFIELD, MBBS, FRACP, PhD
Department of Endocrinology and Diabetes Centre; Diabetes and Obesity Program, Garvan Institute of Medical Research; Faculty of Medicine, University of New South Wales, Sydney, New South Wales, Australia

CAROLINE HAYHURST, MBChB, FRCS
The Centre for Minimally Invasive Neurosurgery, Prince of Wales Private Hospital, Randwick, New South Wales, Australia

KEN K.Y. HO, MD, FRACP
Professor, Centres of Health Research; Department of Diabetes and Endocrinology, Princess Alexandra Hospital; School of Medicine, University of Queensland, Woolloongabba, Brisbane, Queensland, Australia

JOHN Y.K. LEE, MD
Assistant Professor, Department of Neurosurgery, University of Pennsylvania School of Medicine, Hospital of the University of Pennsylvania, Philadelphia, Pennsylvania

PAUL LEE, MBBS, FRACP, PhD
Department of Diabetes and Endocrinology, Princess Alexandra Hospital; School of Medicine, University of Queensland, Woolloongabba, Brisbane, Queensland, Australia

JAMES N. PALMER, MD
Associate Professor, Department of Otorhinolaryngology–Head and Neck Surgery, University of Pennsylvania School of Medicine, Hospital of the University of Pennsylvania, Philadelphia, Pennsylvania

CARLOS D. PINHEIRO-NETO, MD
Department of Otolaryngology, University of Pittsburgh School of Medicine, Pittsburgh, Pennsylvania

J. DREW PROSSER, MD
Resident, Department of Otolaryngology, Medical College of Georgia, Augusta, Georgia

KRISTEN O. RILEY, MD
Assistant Professor of Surgery, Division of Neurological Surgery, University of Alabama at Birmingham, Birmingham, Alabama

DAN ROBINSON, BIT, BCom, MB BS (Hons), FRACS
Department of Otolaryngology–Head and Neck Surgery, Royal Prince Alfred Hospital, University of Sydney, Sydney, New South Wales, Australia

RAYMOND SACKS, MBBCH, FCS (SA) ORL, FRACS, MMed (ORL)
Department of Otolaryngology–Head and Neck Surgery, Concord Hospital, Hornsby Hospital, University of Sydney, Sydney, New South Wales, Australia

RODNEY J. SCHLOSSER, MD
Staff Surgeon, Ralph H. Johnson VAMC and Professor and Chief, Division of Rhinology, Department of Otolaryngology–Head and Neck Surgery, Medical University of South Carolina, Charleston, South Carolina

DHARAMBIR SINGH SETHI, MBBS, FRCSEd
Professor of Otolaryngology, Department of Otorhinolaryngology, Singapore General Hospital, Singapore

CARL H. SNYDERMAN, MD, MBA
Professor, Departments of Otolaryngology and Neurological Surgery, University of Pittsburgh School of Medicine; Co-Director, Center for Cranial Base Surgery, University of Pittsburgh Medical Center, Pittsburgh, Pennsylvania

C. ARTURO SOLARES, MD
Assistant Professor, Co-Director of the Georgia Skull Base Center, Department of Otolaryngology, Medical College of Georgia, Augusta, Georgia

ALDO C. STAMM, MD, PhD
Professor, Department of Otolaryngology–Head and Neck Surgery, Federal University of São Paulo; Director São Paulo ENT Center, Professor Edmundo Vasconcelos Hospital, São Paulo, Brazil

CHARLES TEO, MBBS, FRACS, AM
Conjoint Associate Professor, Department of Neurosurgery, University of New South Wales; Director, Centre for Minimally Invasive Neurosurgery, New South Wales, Australia

WILLIAM ALEX VANDERGRIFT III, MD
Assistant Professor, Department of Neurosciences, Medical University of South Carolina, Charleston, South Carolina

EDUARDO VELLUTINI, MD, PhD
Director DFV Neuro, São Paulo, Brazil

JOHN R. VENDER, MD
Co-Director of the Georgia Skull Base Center, Professor, Vice Chairman, Medical Director of Southeast Gamma Knife Center, Department of Neurosurgery, Medical College of Georgia, Augusta, Georgia

ERIC W. WANG, MD
Clinical Instructor, Division of Rhinology, Department of Otolaryngology–Head and Neck Surgery, Medical University of South Carolina, Charleston, South Carolina

GEOFF WILCSEK, MB BS, FRANZCO
Associate Professor, Oculoplastics Unit, Department of Ophthalmology, The Prince of Wales Hospital, University of New South Wales, Sydney, New South Wales, Australia

BRADFORD A. WOODWORTH, MD
Assistant Professor and James J. Hicks Endowed Chair of Otolaryngology; Associate Scientist, Gregory Fleming James Cystic Fibrosis Research Center, Birmingham, Alabama

Contents

Spontaneous cerebrospinal fluid rhinorrhea represents a distinct clinic entity that is likely a variant of idiopathic intracranial hypertension (IIH). Patients with spontaneous cerebrospinal fluid (CSF) leaks are generally middle-aged obese women with radiographic evidence of skull base defects, associated meningoencephaloceles, and empty sella syndrome, a common sign of increased intracranial pressure. Significant overlap exists in the characteristics of patients with spontaneous CSF leak and IIH. Endoscopic repair of the CSF fistula is the gold standard treatment for this condition, but emerging evidence supports the reduction of CSF pressure as an important adjuvant treatment in this patient population.

This article discusses the epidemiology, diagnosis, and management of traumatic cerebrospinal fluid (CSF) leaks. An overview of traumatic CSF leaks is presented, and both conservative and operative therapies are reviewed. Management decisions are discussed based on the current literature. Controversial clinical topics are addressed, including the use of prophylactic antibiotics and the timing of surgical repair.

Osteomata of the frontal and ethmoid sinuses have traditionally been surgically removed via external approaches. However, endoscopic techniques have increasingly been used for the surgical management of selected cases. Advances in visualization and instrumentation, as well as the excellent access provided by the Draf type 3 procedure, expanded the reach of endoscopes. We describe current limits of endoscopic approaches in the removal of osteomata from the frontal sinus and our algorithms for their management. We believe that the vast majority of frontal sinus osteomata can be managed endoscopically, änd that only significant anterior or extreme infero-lateral extension constitute major limiting factors.

This article reviews the current literature and level-1 evidence of the natural history and the medical and surgical treatment of skull base fibrous dysplasia. The high rate of optic nerve (ON) involvement and the potential risk of visual impairment as a result of nerve compression have led many surgeons to suggest prophylactic decompression of the ON in asymptomatic patients. However, review of the cases reported in the literature reveals that ON decompression surgery is indicated only for patients with visual deficits, whereas asymptomatic patients with radiologic evidence of ON compression are better managed conservatively.

Pathology affecting the orbit and orbital apex is diverse and heterogeneous. Many of the differential pathologies require management in a multidisciplinary team involving both otolaryngology and ophthalmology. This article discusses the differential pathologies. Emphasis has been placed on Graves orbitopathy, traumatic optic neuropathy, and the indications for decompression in each. The differential diagnosis for a lesion within the orbit and orbital apex is diverse. The presentation, investigation, and appropriate management of these conditions is discussed with emphasis on traumatic optic neuropathy and Graves orbitopathy.

Endoscopic pituitary surgery has been gaining wide acceptance as the first-line treatment of most functional pituitary adenomas. This technique has many advantages over traditional procedures, and growing evidence supports its use for endocrine control of functioning tumors. This article reviews data on the different modalities of treatment of functioning pituitary adenomas and compares the results. Endoscopic pituitary surgery controls tumor growth and endocrinopathy as well as or better than other treatment modalities. Complication rates are low and patient recovery is fast. Furthermore, surgery provides a means of achieving prompt decompression of neurologic structures and endocrine remission.

Craniopharyngiomas are rare epithelial tumors arising along the path of the craniopharyngeal duct; therefore, they occur in the sellar or suprasellar regions. These tumors commonly lead to neurologic, endocrinological, or visual symptoms. Radical surgery is the treatment of choice in craniopharyngiomas. The transnasal/transsphenoidal endoscopic approach offers the possibility of removing the tumor without retracting brain and optic pathways, with good results. The rate of cerebrospinal fluid fistula has improved due to the use of vascularized mucosal flaps for cranial base reconstruction.

Tuberculum sellae (TS) meningiomas represent a distinct subgroup of anterior cranial fossa meningiomas with distinctive features. Early visual deterioration with optic canal infiltration occurs because of the site of dural origin. The expanded endonasal transsphenoidal approach and the eyebrow supraorbital craniotomy have been advocated as minimally invasive techniques for TS meningiomas. The authors review the current literature on minimally invasive techniques for TS meningiomas to define visual outcomes, extent of resection, and operative morbidity associated with each approach and highlight pertinent features of individual tumors, which favor either a cranial or an endonasal approach to achieve optimal outcomes.

Meningiomas are slow-growing benign tumors believed to originate from arachnoidal cap cells. This article discusses the surgical approaches for resection, especially the transnasal endoscopic approach. Alternative treatment options are primarily used where patients are not surgical candidates or location of recurrence precludes additional surgery. These options include radiotherapy, stereotactic radiosurgery, and chemotherapy. In addition, we discuss the current on going research in molecular targeting agents for meningioma treatment.

Midline congenital lesions are rare and commonly comprise nasal dermoids (NDs), encephaloceles, and gliomas. This article discusses the epidemiology of NDs. Management is also discussed, as well as prognosis.

Juvenile nasopharyngeal angiofibromas (JNAs) are rare, benign, highly vascular, locally aggressive tumors that primarily affect male adolescents. Historical treatment of these neoplasms has been primarily surgical. In the past decade, endoscopic resection of JNAs has become a viable and promising surgical treatment option. Endoscopic resection has many advantages over traditional open techniques, including better cosmesis, decreased blood loss, shortened hospital stays, and equivalent or improved recurrence rates. Emerging endoscopic technology continues to push the boundaries of resection of skull base tumors and will no doubt become the surgical treatment of choice for most JNAs in the near future.

In this article the epidemiology, pathophysiology, clinical presentation, investigation, management, and prognosis of hypopituitarism and hypothalamic dysfunction, arising from skull base pathologies and treatment of these conditions, are reviewed and discussed. The clinical question: "What is the consequence of pituitary hypofunction in young patients (ie, craniopharyngioma)?" is answered based on information provided in the review.

FORTHCOMING ISSUES

Telehealth in Otolaryngology
Michael Holtel, MD, and
Yehudah Roth, MD,
Guest Editors

Cochlear Implants
J. Thomas Roland, MD, and
David Haynes, MD, *Guest Editors*

Vestibular Schwannoma
Fred Telischi, MD, and
Jacques Morcos, MD,
Guest Editors

**Pediatric Otolaryngology Challenges
in Multi-System Disease**
Austin Rose, MD, *Guest Editor*

RECENT ISSUES

Allergies for the Otolaryngologist
B.J. Ferguson, MD, and
Suman Golla, MD, *Guest Editors*
June 2011

Dizziness and Vertigo across the Lifespan
Bradley W. Kesser, MD, and
A. Tucker Gleason, PhD, *Guest Editors*
April 2011

Oral Medicine
Vincent D. Eusterman, MD, DDS, and
Arlen Meyers, MD, MBA, *Guest Editors*
February 2010

RELATED INTEREST ARTICLE

In Neuroimaging Clinics, August 2009
Skull Base and Temporal Bone Imaging
Vincent Fook-Hin Chong, MBBS, MBA, FAMS, *Guest Editor*

THE CLINICS ARE NOW AVAILABLE ONLINE!

Access your subscription at:
www.theclinics.com

Skull Base: Meeting Place for Multidisciplinary Collaboration

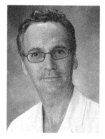 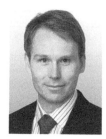

Carl H. Snyderman, MD, MBA   Richard J. Harvey, MD
Guest Editors

The skull base is at a crossroads. It is a meeting point for anatomical regions, surgical specialties, and surgical philosophies. Skull base surgery is a dynamic subspecialty and the last decade has witnessed the application of endoscopic techniques to the ventral skull base using an endonasal corridor. The transition from external approaches to an endonasal corridor has not been without controversy. In this volume, we explore the nascent field of *neurorhinology*, a term that emphasizes the multidisciplinary collaboration between neurosurgeons and rhinologic head and neck surgeons. A wide variety of topics are covered, demonstrating the breadth of skull base surgery.

Neurorhinology has been separated into two volumes, the first volume broadly on the common pathologies encountered and the second volume on more complex lesions. There is a contribution by endocrinologists and radiation oncologists in each issue, respectively. Skill acquisition and training is addressed in the second volume.

We confront the controversies head on, asking the authors to apply evidence-based medicine techniques to critically evaluate the literature and attempt to answer some of the most important clinical questions. We include here portions of the Oxford Centre Evidence-based medicine levels of evidence that were used throughout every discussion (**Tables 1** and **2**). We further hope that the questions raised here will identify areas in need of better data and stimulate new investigations.

As always, we wish to acknowledge our spouses and families, whose support has been an integral part of our careers.

Otolaryngol Clin N Am 44 (2011) xi–xii
doi:10.1016/j.otc.2011.07.001
0030-6665/11/$ – see front matter © 2011 Elsevier Inc. All rights reserved.

oto.theclinics.com

Table 1
The Oxford Centre for Evidence-based Medicine—levels of evidence

Level	Therapy/Prevention/Etiology/Harm
1a	Systematic review (with homogeneity) of randomized controlled trials
1b	Individual randomized controlled trial (with narrow CI)
1c	All or none[a]
2a	Systematic review (with homogeneity) of cohort studies
2b	Individual cohort study (including low-quality randomized controlled trials; eg, <80% follow-up)
2c	"Outcomes" research; ecological studies
3a	Systematic review (with homogeneity) of case-control studies
3b	Individual case-control studies
4	Case-series (and poor-quality cohort and case-control studies)
5	Expert opinion without explicit critical appraisal, or based on physiology, bench research or "first principles"

[a] Met when all patients died before the treatment became available, but now some survive on it; or when some patients died before the treatment became available, but now none die on it.

Adapted from Phillips B, Ball C, Sackett D, et al. Oxford Centre for Evidence-based Medicine—levels of evidence (March 2009). Available at: http://www.cebm.net/index.aspx?o=1025. Accessed November 25, 2010; with permission.

Table 2
The Oxford Centre for Evidence-based Medicine—grades of recommendation

A	Consistent level 1 studies
B	Consistent level 2 or 3 studies or extrapolations from level 1 studies
C	Level 4 studies or extrapolations from level 2 or 3 studies
D	Level 5 studies or troublingly inconsistent or inconclusive studies of any level

Adapted from Phillips B, Ball C, Sackett D, et al. Oxford Centre for Evidence-based Medicine—levels of evidence (March 2009). Available at: http://www.cebm.net/index.aspx?o=1025. Accessed November 25, 2010; with permission.

Carl H. Snyderman, MD, MBA
Departments of Otolaryngology and Neurological Surgery
University of Pittsburgh School of Medicine
Center for Cranial Base Surgery
University of Pittsburgh Medical Center
200 Lothrop Street
Pittsburgh, PA 15213, USA

Richard J. Harvey, MD
University of New South Wales/Macquarie University
Department of Otolaryngology/Skull Base Surgery
St Vincent's Hospital
354 Victoria Street
Sydney, NSW 2010, Australia

E-mail addresses:
snydermanch@upmc.edu (C.H. Snyderman)
richard@sydneyentclinic.com (R.J. Harvey)

Spontaneous CSF Leaks

Eric W. Wang, MD[a], William Alex Vandergrift III, MD[b],
Rodney J. Schlosser, MD[a],*

KEYWORDS

- Spontaneous CSF leak • Idiopathic intracranial hypertension
- Endoscopic CSF repair

EBM Question	Level of Evidence	Grade of Recommendation
Does spontaneous CSF leaks represent a distinct clinical entity and a variant of idiopathic intracranial hypertension?	2b	B
Does a reduction in CSF pressure alone lead to resolution of CSF leaks?	5	D
Does decreasing ICP, transiently or long-term, improve outcomes of endoscopic closure of spontaneous CSF leaks?	4	C

Spontaneous nasal cerebrospinal fluid (CSF) leaks likely represent a distinct clinical entity in which CSF rhinorrhea occurs in the absence of any inciting event. Historically, the term spontaneous CSF leaks included CSF leaks of multiple causes such as delayed CSF leaks after trauma, congenital skull base malformations, and skull base defects from tumors.[1,2] By separating CSF leaks with a discernable cause, spontaneous CSF leaks can be uniformly evaluated and studied. Most of these patients show clinical signs and radiographic features of increased intracranial pressure (ICP).[3,4] Accurately diagnosing patients with spontaneous CSF leaks is critical for the successful repair of these patients because multiple studies have identified increased ICP as a negative risk factor for successful repair.[5-8] Although repair of nasal CSF leaks using endoscopic techniques has high success rates,[9-11] patients

Financial disclosures: None (E.W.W.).
[a] Division of Rhinology, Department of Otolaryngology-Head and Neck Surgery, Medical University of South Carolina, 135 Rutledge Avenue, MSC 550, Charleston, SC 29403, USA
[b] Department of Neurosciences, Medical University of South Carolina, 96 Jonathan Lucas Street, CSB 428, Charleston, SC, USA
* Corresponding author.
E-mail address: schlossr@musc.edu

Otolaryngol Clin N Am 44 (2011) 845–856
doi:10.1016/j.otc.2011.06.018
0030-6665/11/$ – see front matter. Published by Elsevier Inc.

with spontaneous CSF leaks have historically had a significantly lower success rate.[1,3,4,12] This may be explained, in part, by the strong association between spontaneous CSF leaks and idiopathic intracranial hypertension (IIH), a disease associated with increased ICP without other cause. This article examines the evidence correlating spontaneous CSF leaks and IIH and the role of decreasing ICP in the treatment of spontaneous CSF leaks.

NORMAL CSF PHYSIOLOGY

Understanding normal CSF physiology is useful in diagnosing and treating patients with CSF rhinorrhea. CSF is produced in the choroid plexus within the lateral, third, and fourth ventricles at a rate of 0.35 mL/min. CSF is produced by the choroid plexus and flows from the ventricular system into the subarachnoid space. CSF absorption occurs at the arachnoid villi along the cerebral convexities. The villi project into the dural sinuses and act as one-way valves that typically require a pressure gradient of 1.5 to 7 cm H_2O for antegrade flow. At lower pressure differentials, the villi close, preventing retrograde flow. The total volume of CSF in adults is approximately 90 to 150 mL and is turned over 3 to 5 times daily.[13]

Normal CSF pressure is between 5 and 15 cm H_2O in the lumbar cistern with the patient lying in the decubitus position. The pressure varies depending on the time of day, patient age, activity level, and cardiopulmonary cycles. Neurologic symptoms can occur when ICP exceeds 15 to 20 cm H_2O.[13]

CLINICAL PRESENTATION AND EVALUATION OF SPONTANEOUS CSF LEAK

Patients are generally obese middle-aged women who present with spontaneous clear rhinorrhea. Although men and normal-weight women may also present with similar symptoms, the incidence is much lower. The initial diagnostic step is to confirm the presence of CSF in the clear rhinorrhea by laboratory testing. In the United States, β-2 transferrin is the most commonly used laboratory test to confirm the presence of CSF. Cerebral neuraminidase produces β-2 transferrin from β-1 transferrin by desialization. β-2 Transferrin is only found in CSF, perilymph, and the vitreous humor of the eye.[14] The identification of β-2 transferrin in nasal secretions is highly sensitive and specific for CSF rhinorrhea.[15]

After diagnosing CSF rhinorrhea by β-2 transferrin, localization of the skull base defect and site of CSF fistula follows. High-resolution computed tomography (CT) is the initial radiographic test of choice, allowing for evaluation of the bony integrity of the skull base and paranasal sinuses. Patients with spontaneous CSF leaks have characteristic CT findings that support the diagnosis. The bone of the skull base is broadly attenuated and thin.[16] Arachnoid pits secondary to the bony impressions from the arachnoid villi in the skull base are present in 63% of patients with spontaneous CSF leaks.[17] The most common sites of skull base dehiscence are the lateral recess of the sphenoid and the ethmoid roof (**Figs. 1** and **2**).[4,18,19] Pneumatization of the lateral recess of the sphenoid is reported in 91% of patients with spontaneous CSF leaks, in comparison with 23% to 43% in normal patients.[17,20] Dehiscence of the ethmoid roof or cribiform plate is seen in 14% of patients with spontaneous CSF leaks.[21] The presence of multiple skull base defects is common and may be present in 31% of these patients.[19]

Magnetic resonance imaging (MRI) is a useful adjunct in the evaluation of patients with CSF rhinorrhea. Patients with spontaneous CSF leaks have the highest rate of meningoencephalocele formation, ranging from 50% to 100%.[1,11] MRI is effective in assessing the contents of meningoencephalic sacs. Another benefit of MRI in the

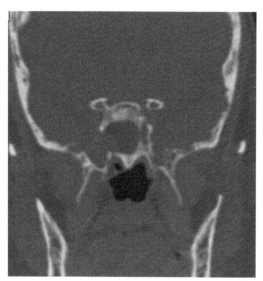

Fig. 1. CT of a meningoencephalocele of the lateral recess of the sphenoid. The skull base bony defect is present in the roof of the sphenoid lateral recess. The skull base is attenuated and arachnoid pits are present. Opacification of the sphenoid sinus with a different density medial to the meningoencephalocele is consistent with CSF filling the remainder of the sphenoid.

evaluation of patients with spontaneous CSF leaks is the recognition of the empty sella. Empty sella syndrome is a common radiographic finding seen in both spontaneous CSF leaks and IIH (**Fig. 3**).[3,19,22] Increased ICP are exerted on sites of inherent structural weakness including the fascia of the sellar diaphragm. The resulting herniation of the meninges and CSF through the sellar diaphragm produces the appearance of an empty sella on MRI. The presence of empty sella syndrome has been associated with both increased ICP and spontaneous CSF leaks.[3] One group has

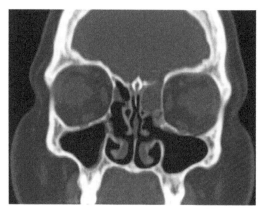

Fig. 2. CT of a spontaneous meningoencephalocele of the ethmoid roof. The skull base defect is small in comparison with the large meningoencephalocele.

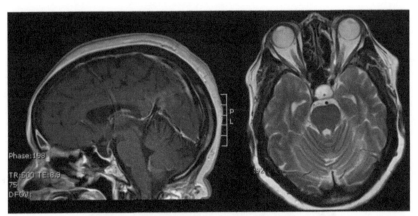

Fig. 3. Empty sella syndrome. Sagittal view of T1 MRI with gadolinium showing fluid filling the sella turcica. The pituitary gland is compressed and not visible. Axial T2 MRI of the same patient showed fluid filling the sella turcica.

suggested that the reversal of empty sella in patients with IIH is a radiographic marker of successful reversal of increased ICP.[22]

Multiple radiographic signs support the theory that spontaneous CSF leaks and IIH are linked. The attenuated skull base with resulting skull base defects, large encephaloceles, and the presence of arachnoid pits support the hypothesis that increased ICPs are contributing to spontaneous CSF leaks. The high prevalence of empty sella syndrome in both IIH and spontaneous CSF leaks further strengthens this correlation.

PATHOPHYSIOLOGY: DO SPONTANEOUS CSF LEAKS REPRESENT A DISTINCT CLINICAL ENTITY AND A VARIANT OF IIH?

Significant overlap exists in the demographic, clinical, and radiographic characteristics of patients with spontaneous CSF leak and IIH. The similarities between these 2 patient populations are striking and strengthen the theory that high-pressure spontaneous CSF leaks are likely a variant of IIH. Patients with IIH classically present with symptoms of headache, pulsatile tinnitus, and visual changes.[23] In case-control trials, factors associated with IIH are female sex, reproductive age, obesity, and recent weight gain.[24,25] Using the modified Dandy criteria to establish the diagnosis of IIH, 70% of patients with spontaneous CSF leaks meet the clinical, radiographic, and ICP criteria for IIH.[26] In addition to clear rhinorrhea, patients often present with pressurelike headaches and pulsatile tinnitus.[26] Case series of patients with spontaneous CSF leaks highlight the overlapping demographics, including female predisposition (70%–80%) and obesity (82%–92%).[12,18,27] Case reports have described patients originally diagnosed with IIH and subsequently presenting with spontaneous CSF rhinorrhea months to years later.[28–30] In most of these patients, the underlying IIH was poorly controlled, suggesting that persistent high intracranial pressure directly resulted in the subsequent CSF rhinorrhea.

The prevalence of obesity in both patient groups is remarkable and may provide some insight into the pathophysiology of both disease processes. For IIH, Radhakrishnan and colleagues[31] calculated an increased incidence of 21.4 per 100,000 for obese women with a body mass index (BMI) of 30, approximately 10-fold to 20-fold higher than the general population. In a large retrospective review of endoscopic CSF leak repair, the average BMI between spontaneous CSF leak (35.4) and traumatic

CSF leak (29.7) was statistically significant.[32] These similarities suggest that obesity has a potential role in the development of spontaneous CSF leaks and further highlights this population as a likely variant of IIH. However, the pathophysiology of both disease processes remains unknown. If the prevalence of obesity is as high as 16%, a higher prevalence of both IIH and spontaneous CSF leaks would be expected if obesity were the primary factor for the development of this condition. Although the recent increased reporting of spontaneous CSF leaks may reflect the increased prevalence of obesity, it seems likely that an additional causal factor or event must be present to develop IIH.

Regardless of the cause of the increased CSF pressure, persistent pulsatile pressure exerted on the skull base at sites of inherent structural weakness results in bony erosion and the potential for CSF leak. Radiographic findings associated with IIH in a blinded case-control study include empty sella syndrome, abnormalities of the optic nerve, arachnoid pits, and skull base flattening, specifically posterior globe flattening.[33] Schlosser and Bolger[3] showed the presence of empty sella syndrome in 100% of patients with multiple spontaneous CSF leaks in comparison with 11% of patients with nonspontaneous CSF leaks. Additional radiographic features seen in spontaneous CSF leaks, such as arachnoid pits, encephaloceles, and dural ectasia, are consistent with increased ICP and support the association with IIH (**Fig. 4**).[34] The presence of skull base fistula and CSF leak in this patient population is not isolated to the anterior cranial fossa. Two retrospective studies of patients with spontaneous CSF otorrhea found an empty sella in 80% of patients as well as similar patient demographics such as increased BMI and female disposition.[35,36]

In addition to these radiographic finding and clinical correlations, direct evidence of increased ICP in patients with spontaneous CSF leak would be expected. In a retrospective analysis evaluating 142 patients with empty sella syndrome, Maira and colleagues[37] found impairment in ICP and CSF dynamics in 76% of patients and 24% of patients were affected by CSF otorrhea. To establish a diagnosis of IIH requires an opening pressure of 25 cm H_2O by lumbar puncture. Prior studies have noted an increased ICP pressures measuring between 27 and 32.5 cm H_2O in patients with spontaneous CSF leak following surgical repair of the leak.[4,12,27] In comparison, a control group of patients with a traumatic CSF leak had a mean postrepair ICP of 14 cm H_2O.[4] The level of ICP pressure in individuals with spontaneous CSF leak is more than normal and consistent with IIH. In addition, these findings suggest that the spontaneous CSF leak may be serving as a release valve, preventing a subset of patients from exhibiting clinical symptoms of IIH until after operative repair.

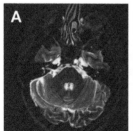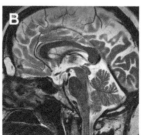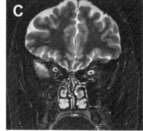

Fig. 4. A patient with spontaneous CSF leak with bilateral petrous meningoceles (*A*), empty sella (*B*) and dilated CSF spaces through the optic nerve sheath (*C*). Such changes highlight the spectrum that these patients might present from benign intracranial hypertension to pseudotumor cerebri.

However, some of the complaints may arise after successful repair if no further intervention to reduce CSF pressure is instituted.[12] No longitudinal studies evaluating the development or persistence of classic IIH symptoms have been performed in patients undergoing successful repair of a spontaneous CSF leak. Prior studies have reported that 31% of patients with spontaneous CSF leaks have multiple skull base defects and are more likely to have multiple encephaloceles, supporting the role of increased ICP in the skull base erosion. In addition, mean ICP in a small set of patients undergoing multiple concurrent skull base repairs for spontaneous CSF leaks was 28.3 cm H_2O.[19] The findings suggest that spontaneous CSF leak is likely a variant of IIH and the increased intracranial pressure in these patients contributes to their CSF leaks.[19]

The current literature on symptom prevalence seen between spontaneous CSF leaks and IIH consists of retrospective cohort studies (level 2B) and case series (level 4). The role for increased ICP in the development of spontaneous CSF leaks includes retrospective cohort trials (level 2B) that support this assertion (grade B recommendation).

MANAGEMENT: DOES A REDUCTION IN CSF PRESSURE ALONE LEAD TO RESOLUTION OF CSF LEAKS?

Ransom and colleagues[38] reported a case of spontaneous CSF leak of the cribiform plate in a patient with IIH after ventriculoperitoneal shunt failure. The patient had no prior history of trauma, sinus surgery, or intracranial surgeries. Successful revision of the ventriculoperitoneal shunt resulted in complete cessation of the CSF rhinorrhea at 1-year follow-up.

The association between obesity and IIH has been reported in multiple studies. In these patients, significant weight loss is associated with a resolution of headache and reduction of CSF pressure. Gastric bypass in these patients reduces CSF pressures from 35.3 ($\pm$3.5) to 16.8 ($\pm$1.2) cm H_2O.[39] At least 3 separate case reports describe the resolution after CSF rhinorrhea after gastric bypass surgery and weight loss.[40–42]

These limited case reports suggesting a decrease of CSF pressure alone for the treatment of CSF rhinorrhea constitute level 5 evidence and a grade D recommendation. However these observations strengthen the contention that IIH contributes to CSF leaks and suggests that decreasing ICP may have a beneficial adjuvant role to endoscopic repair in the management of CSF rhinorrhea.

MANAGEMENT: DOES DECREASING ICP, TRANSIENTLY OR LONG-TERM, IMPROVE OUTCOMES OF ENDOSCOPIC CLOSURE OF SPONTANEOUS CSF LEAKS?

Endonasal endoscopic repair of CSF rhinorrhea is the standard of care and offers the advantages of avoiding the traditional morbidities of a frontal craniotomy, excellent visualization of the skull base defect, and high success rates.[10,43,44] As previously noted, multiple studies have reported a success rate of more than 90% for endoscopic repair in patient series in which most leaks were traumatic or iatrogenic. In the subset of patients with spontaneous CSF leaks, the historical success rate is substantially lower, with recurrences noted in 25% to 87% of patients.[1,2,6,11,16] Recent studies suggest that control of increased ICP can improve success rates in patients with spontaneous CSF leaks equivalent to those of other causes.[5,27]

Operative techniques for endonasal endoscopic CSF leak closure are described in detail in other publications by the senior author.[45] Because of the high incidence of recurrence, additional precautions should be undertaken in the repair of spontaneous CSF leaks. Reduction of the meningoencephalocele with bipolar cautery should be undertaken with meticulous care to avoid intracranial bleeds. With small defects, a reduction in the encephalocele and an overlay graft, either free or pedicled, may be adequate. In larger defects, the placement of an underlay bone graft is believed to provide additional structural support to skull base repairs in cases with increased ICP. Great care should be taken in the shaping and placement of this underlay bone graft because the skull base in spontaneous CSF leaks is broadly attenuated and may fracture easily.[45] A variety of overlay graft materials have been shown to be effective and the specific graft material chosen is dependent on the size, location, and shape of the defect and on the surgeon's preference.

Specific postoperative concerns related to the increased ICP in patients with spontaneous CSF leaks exist. Once the CSF fistula is closed, ICP tends to increase because CSF diversion into the nasal cavity no longer exists. Prior studies have noted increased ICP pressures measuring between 27 and 32.5 cm H_2O in patients with spontaneous CSF leak following surgical repair of the leak.[4,12,27] This increased ICP may place additional stress on the repair and compromise the successful closure of the fistula. To date, no randomized control trials examining the role of decreasing ICP in patients undergoing CSF fistula closure were identified. Two large retrospective studies have used lumbar drains to reduce increased ICP in patients with high-pressure CSF leaks with increased success rates and to determine which patients require long-term management of ICP.[5,27]

Lumbar drains have been advocated to transiently reduce CSF pressure in the immediate postoperative period and may serve to determine which patients require long-term management of increased ICP. Carrau and colleagues[5] reported on 19 patients with high-pressure CSF leaks undergoing CSF fistula repair and using a lumbar drain in the immediate postoperative period to reduce CSF pressure. If persistently increased ICPs were noted after the repair, the patients underwent immediate ventriculoperitoneal shunt placement. The success rate was 100%, with a mean follow-up of 30 months. This study also supports decreasing ICP in all patients with high-pressure CSF leak, including spontaneous CSF rhinorrhea and subarachnoid hemorrhage. Woodworth and colleagues[27] reported on 77 patients with spontaneous CSF leaks who underwent skull base repair. Lumbar drains were used in all patients and, if CSF pressure were increased (>15 cm H_2O) on postoperative day 2, medical therapy with acetazolamide was initiated. Patients with significantly increased ICP (>35 cm H_2O) were recommended to have a ventriculoperitoneal shunt. Using this protocol, the success rate in this case-control study was 89%, with a mean follow-up of 30 months. A closer examination of the patient who failed in this trial further supports the contention that successful CSF fistula closure rates are improved by lowering ICP. In the 6 patients who had recurrent CSF leak, 3 patients failed at a new distant site. The investigators considered this a failure of management of ICP, rather than a technical error. In addition, 3 patients who failed had increased ICP secondary to shunt failure.[27] Other studies have disputed the need for lumbar drains in the postoperative period, reporting a 97% success rate without the use of lumbar drain and no other management of ICP.[46] However, the number of patients with spontaneous CSF leak in this case series is limited (4/33), thus preventing accurate comparisons.

Multiple investigators have advocated the routine use of acetazolamide in all patients with spontaneous CSF leaks and evidence of increased CSF pressure.[4,7] Acetazolamide lowers CSF production by 48%.[47] Prior studies have shown a mean reduction of 10 cm H_2O in CSF pressure with the institution of acetazolamide in addition to a decrease in pressurelike headache and pulsatile tinnitus.[4] Despite the objective reduction in CSF pressure and the increased success of endoscopic repair of high-pressure CSF fistula with adjuvant therapy to reduce CSF pressure, the long-term benefit remains unproven and it is unlikely that prospective controlled trials will be conducted.

Interventions to reduce ICP have been more extensively studied in patients with IIH, but there is insufficient evidence on which to base treatment of IIH. A recent Cochrane systematic review of interventions for IIH identified 7 studies related to the treatment of IIH, but no randomized trials were found.[23] The investigators concluded that there are insufficient data to determine an evidence-based management strategy for IIH. Although acetazolamide is frequently used as the initial therapy for IIH, the studies are conflicting regarding its efficacy in reducing visual symptoms. Using visual field improvement as the primary outcome measure, acetazolamide was effective in the treatment of IIH in a 12-month period.[48] In contrast, a prospective cohort trial concluded that acetazolamide alone was ineffective in reducing papilledema.[49] In addition to acetazolamide, recent reports also suggest the efficacy of topiramate in the treatment of IIH. Topiramate is licensed for the treatment of epilepsy and migraine prevention, but is used off label for other indications. Similar to acetazolamide, topiramate is also a carbonic anhydrase inhibitor and this may represent its mechanism of action in reducing CSF pressure.[50] A recent open-label randomized trial comparing the efficacy of topiramate and acetazolamide concluded that both medications were effective in the treatment of IIH, but topiramate had the added benefit of weight reduction.[48] Acetazolamide is commonly used in the treatment of spontaneous CSF leaks and IIH to reduce ICP. Although the efficacy of acetazolamide in improving success rates after endoscopic closure is supported by case series trials, no randomized control trials in either the spontaneous CSF leak or IIH literature were found.

There is no clear consensus regarding the role of CSF diversion procedures in the repair of spontaneous CSF leaks. As previously noted, Carrau and collegues[5] recommended immediate VP shunting procedures in all patients with high-pressure CSF leaks. Woodworth and colleagues[27] recommended CSF shunting in patients with ICP greater than 35 cm H_2O after closure. In a large retrospective analysis of patients with empty sella syndrome, CSF shunting procedures were found to be effective in reducing neurologic symptoms, improving vision, and aiding the repair of CSF rhinorrhea.[37] In a recent systematic review of surgical interventions for IIH to reduce visual symptoms, the investigators concluded that both lumbar peritoneal shunting and ventriculoperitoneal shunting are effective in preventing visual loss.[51] However, both interventions were noted to fail in a proportion of patients and to have associated complications. Curry and colleagues[52] reviewed the population data from 1988 to 2002 for CSF shunting procedures for IIH and found that 54% of patients had a lumbo-peritoneal shunt, 39% had a ventriculoperitoneal shunt, and 2% had both. The most significant determining factor for which procedure was chosen was the geographic state. The role of CSF diversion in both spontaneous CSF leaks and IIH requires further study. CSF diversion is effective in reducing ICP, but associated comorbidities, including the need for revisions of the shunt, require the careful consideration of the risk/benefit ratio in a given patient. At present, the long-term benefit of decreased ICP in patients with spontaneous CSF leak, either via medications, weight loss, or CSF diversion, is not clearly defined, although case series trials generally support the use of these strategies.

The level of evidence supporting the use of medications or CSF diversion procedures in the treatment of spontaneous CSF leaks is level 4 and constitutes a grade C recommendation. The trials are solely retrospective case series with no controls (**Table 1**).

Table 1
Grade of evidence correlating spontaneous CSF leaks and IIH and the role of decreasing ICP in the treatment of spontaneous CSF leaks

Evidenced-based Question	Grade of Evidence
Association between IIH and spontaneous CSF leaks: demographic, clinical presentation, radiographic findings	B
Etiologic role of increased ICP in spontaneous CSF leaks	B
Decreasing ICP alone for the treatment of spontaneous CSF leak	D
Improving outcomes after endoscopic repair of CSF leaks by decreasing ICP through medication or CSF shunting	C

Abbreviations: ICP, intracranial pressure; IIH, idiopathic intracranial hypertension.

SUMMARY

Spontaneous CSF leak is likely a distinct clinical entity that is associated with increased CSF pressures. The association between spontaneous CSF leaks and IIH, a condition defined by increased ICP without clear cause, is strongly supported by strikingly similar demographic, clinical, and radiologic findings noted in retrospective cohort trial and case series (grade B recommendation). Recent case-control trials support the role of decreasing ICP via medication, weight loss, or CSF diversion to improve successful outcomes after endoscopic repair (grade C recommendation).

EBM Question	Author's reply
Do spontaneous CSF leaks represent a distinct clinical entity and a variant of idiopathic intracranial hypertension?	Spontaneous CSF are both associated with raised ICP and idiopathic intracranial hypertension
Does a reduction in CSF pressure alone lead to resolution of CSF leaks?	Case reports describe resolution of CSF leaks with both diversion and other methods of CSF pressure reduction.
Does decreasing ICP, transiently or long-term, improve outcomes of endoscopic closure of spontaneous CSF leaks?	CSF pressure modifying medications and diversion have been shown to improve the longterm morbidity of IIH patients.

REFERENCES

1. Hubbard JL, McDonald TJ, Pearson BW, et al. Spontaneous cerebrospinal fluid rhinorrhea: evolving concepts in diagnosis and surgical management based on the Mayo Clinic experience from 1970 through 1981. Neurosurgery 1985;16(3): 314–21.
2. Ommaya AK, Di Chiro G, Baldwin M, et al. Non-traumatic cerebrospinal fluid rhinorrhoea. J Neurol Neurosurg Psychiatry 1968;31(3):214–25.
3. Schlosser RJ, Bolger WE. Significance of empty sella in cerebrospinal fluid leaks. Otolaryngol Head Neck Surg 2003;128(1):32–8.
4. Schlosser RJ, Wilensky EM, Grady MS, et al. Cerebrospinal fluid pressure monitoring after repair of cerebrospinal fluid leaks. Otolaryngol Head Neck Surg 2004; 130(4):443–8.
5. Carrau RL, Snyderman CH, Kassam AB. The management of cerebrospinal fluid leaks in patients at risk for high-pressure hydrocephalus. Laryngoscope 2005; 115(2):205–12.

6. Mirza S, Thaper A, McClelland L, et al. Sinonasal cerebrospinal fluid leaks: management of 97 patients over 10 years. Laryngoscope 2005;115(10):1774–7.

7. Woodworth BA, Palmer JN. Spontaneous cerebrospinal fluid leaks. Curr Opin Otolaryngol Head Neck Surg 2009;17(1):59–65.

8. Basu D, Haughey BH, Hartman JM. Determinants of success in endoscopic cerebrospinal fluid leak repair. Otolaryngol Head Neck Surg 2006;135(5):769–73.

9. Gassner HG, Ponikau JU, Sherris DA, et al. CSF rhinorrhea: 95 consecutive surgical cases with long term follow-up at the Mayo Clinic. Am J Rhinol 1999; 13(6):439–47.

10. Mattox DE, Kennedy DW. Endoscopic management of cerebrospinal fluid leaks and cephaloceles. Laryngoscope 1990;100(8):857–62.

11. Schick B, Ibing R, Brors D, et al. Long-term study of endonasal duraplasty and review of the literature. Ann Otol Rhinol Laryngol 2001;110(2):142–7.

12. Schlosser RJ, Wilensky EM, Grady MS, et al. Elevated intracranial pressures in spontaneous cerebrospinal fluid leaks. Am J Rhinol 2003;17(4):191–5.

13. Daube JR, Reagan TJ, Sandok BA. The cerebrospinal fluid system. In: Daube JR, Reagan TJ, Sandok BA, editors. Medical neurosciences: an approach to anatomy, pathology and physiology by systems and levels. Boston: Little Brown; 1986. p. 93–111.

14. Ridley F. The intraocular pressure and drainage of aqueous humor. Br J Exp Pathol 1930;11:214–50.

15. Papadea C, Schlosser RJ. Rapid method for beta2-transferrin in cerebrospinal fluid leakage using an automated immunofixation electrophoresis system. Clin Chem 2005;51(2):464–70.

16. Schlosser RJ, Bolger WE. Nasal cerebrospinal fluid leaks: critical review and surgical considerations. Laryngoscope 2004;114(2):255–65.

17. Shetty PG, Shroff MM, Fatterpekar GM, et al. A retrospective analysis of spontaneous sphenoid sinus fistula: MR and CT findings. AJNR Am J Neuroradiol 2000; 21(2):337–42.

18. Kirtane MV, Gautham K, Upadhyaya SR. Endoscopic CSF rhinorrhea closure: our experience in 267 cases. Otolaryngol Head Neck Surg 2005;132(2):208–12.

19. Schlosser RJ, Bolger WE. Management of multiple spontaneous nasal meningoencephaloceles. Laryngoscope 2002;112(6):980–5.

20. Bolger WE, Butzin CA, Parsons DS. Paranasal sinus bony anatomic variations and mucosal abnormalities: CT analysis for endoscopic sinus surgery. Laryngoscope 1991;101(1 Pt 1):56–64.

21. Ohnishi T. Bony defects and dehiscences of the roof of the ethmoid cells. Rhinology 1981;19(4):195–202.

22. Zagardo MT, Cail WS, Kelman SE, et al. Reversible empty sella in idiopathic intracranial hypertension: an indicator of successful therapy? AJNR Am J Neuroradiol 1996;17(10):1953–6.

23. Lueck CJ, McIlwaine GG. Interventions for idiopathic intracranial hypertension. Cochrane Database Syst Rev 2009;4:1–12 [Review].

24. Giuseffi V, Wall M, Siegel PZ, et al. Symptoms and disease associations in idiopathic intracranial hypertension (pseudotumor cerebri): a case-control study. Neurology 1991;41(2 Pt 1):239–44.

25. Ireland B, Corbett JJ, Wallace RB. The search for causes of idiopathic intracranial hypertension. A preliminary case-control study. Arch Neurol 1990;47(3):315–20.

26. Schlosser RJ, Woodworth BA, Wilensky EM, et al. Spontaneous cerebrospinal fluid leaks: a variant of benign intracranial hypertension. Ann Otol Rhinol Laryngol 2006;115(7):495–500.

27. Woodworth BA, Prince A, Chiu AG, et al. Spontaneous CSF leaks: a paradigm for definitive repair and management of intracranial hypertension. Otolaryngol Head Neck Surg 2008;138(6):715–20.
28. Camras LR, Ecanow JS, Abood CA. Spontaneous cerebrospinal fluid rhinorrhea in a patient with pseudotumor cerebri. J Neuroimaging 1998;8(1):41–2.
29. Clark D, Bullock P, Hui T, et al. Benign intracranial hypertension: a cause of CSF rhinorrhoea. J Neurol Neurosurg Psychiatry 1994;57(7):847–9.
30. Owler BK, Allan R, Parker G, et al. Pseudotumour cerebri, CSF rhinorrhoea and the role of venous sinus stenting in treatment. Br J Neurosurg 2003;17(1):79–83.
31. Radhakrishnan K, Thacker AK, Bohlaga NH, et al. Epidemiology of idiopathic intracranial hypertension: a prospective and case-control study. J Neurol Sci 1993;116(1):18–28.
32. Banks CA, Palmer JN, Chiu AG, et al. Endoscopic closure of CSF rhinorrhea: 193 cases over 21 years. Otolaryngol Head Neck Surg 2009;140(6):826–33.
33. Agid R, Farb RI, Willinsky RA, et al. Idiopathic intracranial hypertension: the validity of cross-sectional neuroimaging signs. Neuroradiology 2006;48(8):521–7.
34. Silver RI, Moonis G, Schlosser RJ, et al. Radiographic signs of elevated intracranial pressure in idiopathic cerebrospinal fluid leaks: a possible presentation of idiopathic intracranial hypertension. Am J Rhinol 2007;21(3):257–61.
35. Goddard JC, Meyer T, Nguyen S, et al. New considerations in the cause of spontaneous cerebrospinal fluid otorrhea. Otol Neurotol 2010;31(6):940–5.
36. Kutz JW Jr, Husain IA, Isaacson B, et al. Management of spontaneous cerebrospinal fluid otorrhea. Laryngoscope 2008;118(12):2195–9.
37. Maira G, Anile C, Mangiola A. Primary empty sella syndrome in a series of 142 patients. J Neurosurg 2005;103(5):831–6.
38. Ransom ER, Komotar RJ, Mocco J, et al. Shunt failure in idiopathic intracranial hypertension presenting with spontaneous cerebrospinal fluid leak. J Clin Neurosci 2006;13(5):598–602.
39. Sugerman HJ, Felton WL 3rd, Salvant JB Jr, et al. Effects of surgically induced weight loss on idiopathic intracranial hypertension in morbid obesity. Neurology 1995;45(9):1655–9.
40. Rudnick E, Sismanis A. Pulsatile tinnitus and spontaneous cerebrospinal fluid rhinorrhea: indicators of benign intracranial hypertension syndrome. Otol Neurotol 2005;26(2):166–8.
41. Stangherlin P, Ledeghen S, Scordidis V, et al. Benign intracranial hypertension with recurrent spontaneous cerebrospinal fluid rhinorrhoea treated by laparoscopic gastric banding. Acta Chir Belg 2008;108(5):616–8.
42. Sugerman HJ, Felton WL 3rd, Sismanis A, et al. Gastric surgery for pseudotumor cerebri associated with severe obesity. Ann Surg 1999;229(5):634–40 [discussion: 640–2].
43. Hegazy HM, Carrau RL, Snyderman CH, et al. Transnasal endoscopic repair of cerebrospinal fluid rhinorrhea: a meta-analysis. Laryngoscope 2000;110(7):1166–72.
44. Lanza DC, O'Brien DA, Kennedy DW. Endoscopic repair of cerebrospinal fluid fistulae and encephaloceles. Laryngoscope 1996;106(9 Pt 1):1119–25.
45. Schlosser RJ, Bolger WE. Endoscopic management of cerebrospinal fluid rhinorrhea. Otolaryngol Clin North Am 2006;39(3):523–38, ix.
46. Casiano RR, Jassir D. Endoscopic cerebrospinal fluid rhinorrhea repair: is a lumbar drain necessary? Otolaryngol Head Neck Surg 1999;121(6):745–50.
47. Carrion E, Hertzog JH, Medlock MD, et al. Use of acetazolamide to decrease cerebrospinal fluid production in chronically ventilated patients with ventriculopleural shunts. Arch Dis Child 2001;84(1):68–71.

48. Celebisoy N, Gokcay F, Sirin H, et al. Treatment of idiopathic intracranial hypertension: topiramate vs acetazolamide, an open-label study. Acta Neurol Scand 2007;116(5):322–7.

49. Johnson LN, Krohel GB, Madsen RW, et al. The role of weight loss and acetazolamide in the treatment of idiopathic intracranial hypertension (pseudotumor cerebri). Ophthalmology 1998;105(12):2313–7.

50. Mirza N, Marson AG, Pirmohamed M. Effect of topiramate on acid-base balance: extent, mechanism and effects. Br J Clin Pharmacol 2009;68(5):655–61.

51. Brazis PW. Clinical review: the surgical treatment of idiopathic pseudotumour cerebri (idiopathic intracranial hypertension). Cephalalgia 2008;28(12):1361–73.

52. Curry WT Jr, Butler WE, Barker FG 2nd. Rapidly rising incidence of cerebrospinal fluid shunting procedures for idiopathic intracranial hypertension in the United States, 1988-2002. Neurosurgery 2005;57(1):97–108 [discussion: 97–108].

Traumatic Cerebrospinal Fluid Leaks

J. Drew Prosser, MD[a], John R. Vender, MD[b],
C. Arturo Solares, MD[a,*]

KEYWORDS

- Cerebrospinal fluid leak • Skull base trauma
- Skull base surgery • CSF rhinorrhea

Key Points: CSF LEAKS

- Eighty percent of cerebrospinal fluid (CSF) leaks occur following nonsurgical trauma and complicate 2% of all head traumas, and 12% to 30% of all basilar skull fractures

- The most common presentation is unilateral watery rhinorrhea, and β_2-transferrin is now the preferred method of confirming a fluid as CSF

- High-resolution computed tomography (CT) is the preferred method of localizing the site of skull base defect following craniomaxillofacial trauma, but can be coupled with magnetic resonance imaging (MRI) or cisternography

- Conservative management of CSF leaks includes strict bed rest, elevation of the head, and avoidance of straining, retching, or nose blowing, and results in resolution of the majority of traumatic CSF leaks over a 7-day period

- CSF diversion improves the rates of resolution when added to conservative therapy

- Endoscopic endonasal approaches should be the preferred method of repair with greater than 90% success rates; however, open transcranial and extracranial repairs still have their place in operative management

- Small postsurgical defects can be repaired endoscopically with mucosal grafts, while the pedicled nasal septal flap has emerged as the preferred method of repair for large defects

- Prophylactic antibiotics have not been shown to reduce the risk of meningitis and may select for more virulent organisms

- Data suggest that early surgical repair (<7 days) can reduce the risk of meningitis.

The authors have no relevant disclosures.

[a] Department of Otolaryngology, Medical College of Georgia, 1120 15th Street, BP 4109, Augusta, GA 30912, USA

[b] Medical Director of Southeast Gamma Knife Center, Department of Neurosurgery, Medical College of Georgia, 1120 15th Street, BI 3088, Augusta, GA 30912, USA

* Corresponding author.

E-mail address: csolares@mcg.edu

Otolaryngol Clin N Am 44 (2011) 857–873
doi:10.1016/j.otc.2011.06.007
0030-6665/11/$ – see front matter © 2011 Elsevier Inc. All rights reserved.

oto.theclinics.com

EBM Question	Level of Evidence	Grade of Recommendation
Do spontaneous CSF leaks represent a distinct clinical entity and a variant of idiopathic intracranial hypertension?	2b	B
Does a reduction in CSF pressure alone lead to resolution of CSF leaks?	5	D
Does decreasing ICP, transiently or long-term, improve outcomes of endoscopic closure of spontaneous CSF leaks?	4	C

CSF is an ultrafiltrate of plasma or serum, which contains electrolytes, glucose, and proteins. Located in the cerebral ventricles and cranial/spinal subarachnoid space, this fluid serves in physical support and provides buoyancy for the brain and spinal elements. CSF also serves to maintain homeostasis of neural tissues by removing by-products of metabolism and regulating the chemical environment of the brain.[1] CSF is produced by the choroid plexus in the lateral, third, and fourth ventricles. It circulates from the lateral ventricles through the foramina of Monro into the third ventricle and then to the fourth ventricle through the aqueduct of Sylvius, then communicates with the subarachnoid space through the foramen of Magendie and foramina of Luschka. CSF circulates throughout the meninges between the arachnoid and is reabsorbed into the venous system via arachnoid villi, which project into the dural venous sinuses. Adults average 140 mL of CSF volume, and the body produces 0.33 mL of CSF per minute and thus regenerates its CSF volume 3 times per day.[1] As CSF is an ultrafiltrate of serum, serum abnormalities will be reflected in CSF (ie, hyperglycemia). Fluctuations in the cerebral blood flow related to the cardiac output result in generalized brain volume fluctuations, which gives rise to the vascular pulsations seen in CSF. In addition, major branches of the circle of Willis are located in the subarachnoid space and are likely contribute to this phenomenon.

CSF leaks are rare but are associated with morbidity such as general malaise and headache. More importantly, they can lead to potentially life-threatening complications such as meningitis. As such, they require thorough and timely evaluation and treatment. CSF leaks occur when the bony cranial vault and its underlying dura are breached. Such leaks may be broadly categorized as traumatic or nontraumatic in origin. Traumatic causes can be further subclassified into surgical and nonsurgical, with surgical causes divided into planned (as in failure of reconstruction of a planned dural resection) or unplanned (as a complication following an ethmoidectomy).[2] Nontraumatic CSF leaks may be subclassified into high or normal pressure leaks, with the recognition that tumors can occupy either subclass by mass effect in the high-pressure group or by direct erosive effect on the skull base in the normal-pressure group. If no cause can be found the leak may be classified as idiopathic; however, with careful history taking, physical examination (including nasal endoscopy), and radiologic evaluation, true idiopathic leaks are rare.[2]

EPIDEMIOLOGY OF CEREBROSPINAL FLUID LEAKS

Approximately 80% of CSF leaks result from nonsurgical trauma, 16% from surgical procedures (although this number is rising), and the remaining 4% are nontraumatic. Of the traumatic leaks, more than 50% are evident within the first 2 days, 70% within the first week, and almost all present within the first 3 months.[3,4] Delayed presentation may result from wound contraction or scar formation, necrosis of bony edges or soft tissue, slow resolution of edema, devascularization of tissues, posttreatment tumor retraction, or progressive increases in intracranial pressure (secondary to brain edema or other process). As with most maxillofacial trauma, traumatic CSF leaks occur most commonly in young males and complicate 2% of all head traumas, and 12% to 30% of all basilar skull fractures.[5]

Anterior skull base leaks are more common than middle or posterior leaks, due to the firm adherence of the dura to the anterior basilar skull. The most common sites of CSF rhinorrhea following accidental trauma are the sphenoid sinus (30%), frontal sinus (30%), and ethmoid/cribriform (23%) (**Fig. 1**).[6] Temporal bone fractures with resultant CSF leak can present with CSF otorrhea or rhinorrhea via egress through the Eustachian tube with an intact tympanic membrane. Although a rare complication of functional endoscopic sinus surgery (FESS), the frequency in which this procedure is performed makes it a significant cause of CSF leaks (**Fig. 2**). When looking at surgical trauma, the most common sites of CSF leak following FESS are ethmoid/cribiform (80%), followed the frontal sinus (8%) and sphenoid sinus (4%). After neurosurgical procedures the most common site of CSF leak is the sphenoid sinus (67%) because of the high number of pituitary tumors that are addressed via transsphenoidal approach.[6]

Regarding nontraumatic leaks, high-pressure leaks comprise approximately half of these, with more than 80% resulting from tumor obstruction.[7] The remainder is caused by either benign intracranial hypertension (BIH) or hydrocephalus; however, recent publications suggest an increased role of BIH in idiopathic or "spontaneous" CSF leaks.[8] One hypothesis is that in patients with occult elevated CSF pressure, an intermittent CSF leak may serve as a release valve that decompresses the elevated pressure. Once the leak resolves, either by the normalization of CSF pressure with an intermittent leak or by surgical repair, the CSF pressure will slowly increase and result in recurrence of the leak. It is not surprising that the association between idiopathic

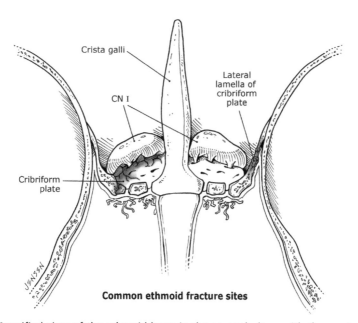

Common ethmoid fracture sites

Fig. 1. Magnified view of the ethmoid bone in the coronal plane with the most common sites of fracture labeled. CN, cranial nerve.

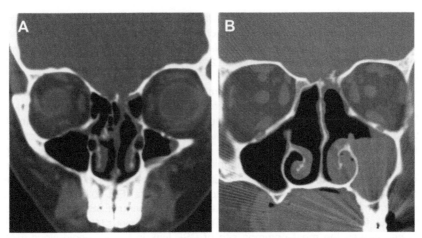

Fig. 2. Coronal CT scan demonstrating a defect in the roof of the left ethmoid sinus (*A*), and a defect in a separate patient with displacement of bony fragments intracranially (*B*). Both are the result of surgical trauma, sustained at another institution.

CSF leaks and BIH has been made, as the demographics of the populations are quite similar.[9] Furthermore, the clinical manifestations and demographic profile of patients with empty sella syndrome are highly similar to those for patients with BIH and patients with nontraumatic CSF leaks.[10] These associations have important clinical implications in the management of idiopathic CSF leaks as well as surgical failures after traumatic CSF leak repair.

DETECTION OF CEREBROSPINAL FLUID LEAKS
Presentation

Presentation of traumatic CSF leaks can be subtle, and diligence is required when one is suspected. Fain and colleagues[11] presented an analysis of 80 cases of trauma to the cranial base. From these cases they determined that there are 5 types of frontobasal trauma. Type I involves only the anterior wall of the frontal sinus. Type II involves the face (craniofacial disjunction of the Lefort II type or crush face), extending upward to the cranial base and to the anterior wall of the frontal sinus, because of the facial retrusion. Type III involves the frontal part of the skull and extends down to the cranial base. Type IV is a combination of types II and III, whereas type V involves only ethmoid or sphenoid bones. In this study CSF leaks were infrequent in types I and II, but occurred more frequently in types III, IV, and V, which included a dural tear in each case. Therefore, when a patient presents with one of these fractures a CSF leak should be suspected.

The most common presenting sign is unilateral watery rhinorrhea following skull base trauma. Patients may complain of a salty or even sweet taste in their mouth; however, with severe trauma to the skull, history may be unobtainable secondary to the patient's neurologic status. Rhinorrhea is classically positional in nature and is most commonly associated with standing or leaning forward. Although this presentation seems straightforward, establishment of the diagnosis and precise localization of the leak can present major challenges. Other rhinologic pathology, including seasonal allergic rhinitis, perennial nonallergic rhinitis, and vasomotor rhinitis, are relatively common, and may mimic some of the signs and symptoms of CSF rhinorrhea or may occur simultaneously with a CSF leak. Furthermore, CSF rhinorrhea is often intermittent, even after trauma, which may lead to false-negative results on diagnostic testing if testing is performed during the quiescent phase. Lastly, the subarachnoid cistern is a relatively low-pressure system. Thus, leaks may be of low volume, which can lead to false-negative testing or failure to recognize that a leak even exists. In cases of high clinical suspicion and initially negative diagnostic testing, further follow-up with repeat testing is warranted.

Identification

Traditionally the presence of a halo sign (clear ring surrounding a central bloody spot) on gauze, tissue, or linen has been used to predict CSF leak following trauma. This halo forms as blood and CSF separate; however, this test should only be used to arouse suspicion as tears, saliva, and other non-CSF rhinorrhea can give false-positive results. Historically the components of the rhinorrhea (including glucose, protein, and electrolytes) have been measured to confirm the diagnosis of CSF. These tests, however, should not be relied on, as their sensitivity and specificity are unacceptably low.[7,12,13]

β_2-Transferrin has emerged as a highly sensitive and specific way of identifying CSF, and is now the preferred method of confirming a fluid as CSF. The method was initially discovered in 1979 by Meurman and colleagues[14] who, when performing protein electrophoresis of CSF, tears, nasal secretions, and serum, noted a β_2-transferrin fraction only in the CSF samples. Techniques for isolating this marker have been subsequently simplified and refined, leading to enhanced sensitivity and specificity.[15,16] As with any test, a reliable result requires an adequate sample. Of note, although quite specific, there are reports of β_2-transferrin being detected in aqueous humor[17] and in the serum of patients with alcohol-related chronic liver disease.[18]

Beta-trace protein (βTP) is another marker that has been used for the detection of CSF. This protein is produced by the meninges and choroid plexus and is released into CSF. It is present in other body fluids, including serum, but at much lower concentrations than in CSF. Detection of βTP has 100% sensitivity and specificity in cases of confirmed CSF rhinorrhea, but cannot be reliably used in patients with renal insufficiency or bacterial meningitis, because serum and CSF levels of βTP substantially increase with reduced glomerular filtration rate and decrease with bacterial meningitis.[19,20]

LOCALIZATION

Once confirmed, localization of the dural defect is critical to management of CSF leaks, particularly if operative management is considered. Following identification of a traumatic CSF leak, nasal endoscopy should be performed. This procedure may narrow the side/site of the leak. Findings commonly are nonspecific, including glistening of nasal mucosa, but occasionally active leaks can be identified. Although direct visualization plays an important role, imaging of the skull base is critical to localization of CSF leaks, particularly traumatic leaks.

High-Resolution CT Scan

Multiple imaging studies have been used to localize defects, but the most common is high-resolution CT (HRCT) scanning. This technology uses 1- to 2-mm sections in both the coronal and axial planes with bone algorithm (see **Fig. 2**), resulting in localization of the majority of skull base defects that result in CSF leak. However, it is important to recognize that congenital or acquired thinning or absence of portions of the bony skull base may be identified and may not necessarily correspond to the site of CSF leak.[21]

This technology can be used with most surgical image guidance systems. Due to the relative ease of obtaining this study and high degree of accuracy, this method should be used as the primary imaging modality for traumatic CSF leaks. Plain CT scans may lead to false-positive results secondary to volume averaging, and their use should be limited. The use of intrathecal fluorescein in combination with HRCT allows for the identification of most CSF leaks.

Intrathecal Fluorescein

Intrathecal agents have been used both to confirm the presence of and to attempt to localize CSF leaks. These agents are administered via lumbar puncture into the subarachnoid space and, as such, complications can be severe. Visible dyes, radioopaque dyes, and radioactive markers have been used with a positive result being visualization, either directly or radiographically, of the agent within the nose and paranasal sinuses.

Intrathecal fluorescein is the most popular visible agent. Popularized by Messerklinger,[22] intrathecal fluorescein has been associated with multiple complications, including grand mal seizures and even death. However, in a study of 420 administrations low-dose (50 mg or less) intrathecal fluorescein was found to be useful in localizing CSF fistulas and was deemed unlikely to be associated with adverse events, as most complications were dose-related.[23] The current recommended dilution is 0.1 mL of 10% intravenous fluorescein (not ophthalmic preparation) in 10 mL of the patient's own CSF, which is infused slowly over 30 minutes. Patients should be extensively counseled about the risks, as this use is not approved by the US Food and Drug Administration (ie, off-label use).

CT Cisternograms

CT cisternography involves the intrathecal administration of radiopaque contrast (metrizamide, iohexol, or iopamidol) followed by CT scanning. Studies have shown that approximately 80% of CSF leaks can be confirmed through this technology.[20] Weaknesses of this technology include its invasive nature, which can limit its use particularly in the pediatric population, as well as its low sensitivity in intermittent leaks.[24] Positive findings usually reveal pooling of contrast in the frontal or sphenoid sinuses, but may not necessarily locate the actual defect. Furthermore, the density of the dye may obscure bony anatomy, leading to more difficulty in locating the bony defect.

Radionuclide Cisternograms

A variety of radioactive markers have been used to detect CSF leaks, including radioactive iodine (^{131}I)-labeled serum albumin, technetium (^{99m}Tc)-labeled serum albumin or diethylenetriamine penta-acetic acid (DTPA), and radioactive indium (^{111}In)-labeled DTPA. This technique is similar to intrathecal fluorescein and involves administration of the tracer via a lumbar puncture. Intranasal pledgets are placed in defined locations under endoscopic guidance and analyzed for tracer uptake approximately 12 to 24 hours later. A scintillation camera is also used, but has poor resolution and difficulty precisely localizing the leak. Overpressure radionuclide cisternography increases the intrathecal pressure with a constant infusion to improve the sensitivity of radionuclide cisternography[25]; however, this modality in clinical practice results in a high degree of false-positive findings with sensitivities from 62% to 76%, limiting its utility.[24]

MRI and MR Cisternograms

In contrast to the previously discussed cisternograms, MR cisternography is a noninvasive method for assessing the presence of intranasal CSF. This technique uses

T2-weighted images with fat suppression and image reversal to highlight CSF. The characteristic signal tracking from the intracranial space to the paranasal sinuses represents a CSF leak. The sensitivity of this test is reported to be 85% to 92%, with 100% specificity.[26] MRI and MR cisternography are able to distinguish inflammatory tissue from meningoencephaloceles; however, bony detail is poor (**Fig. 3**).

Cisternography warrants discussion however, because of the specificity and noninvasive nature of β_2-transferrin testing, the role of various cisternography studies has been significantly altered. In the authors' practice, after the diagnosis of a CSF leak has been confirmed through β_2-transferrin testing, high-resolution CT and MRI of the skull base are used to detail the anatomic integrity of the skull base. Endoscopic exploration confirms the location and is used for repair of the defect (discussed later) in the majority of cases. This philosophy has been adopted by other investigators as well.[27] Using this approach CT and MRI are complementary studies, with CT providing detailed bony anatomy, particularly skull base dehiscence/fractures, and MRI providing soft-tissue detail, including coincident meningoencephaloceles and incidental intracranial pathology. Modern image-guidance software enables the application of CT-MRI fusion for surgical navigation, and results in accurately identifying and localizing the site of CSF leakage in 90% of cases.[28]

CONSERVATIVE MANAGEMENT

Once a CSF leak has been confirmed and localized, the optimal management decision depends on a variety of factors. Even if the otolaryngologist is primarily managing the CSF leak, direct input should be obtained from the trauma service, neurosurgical team and, particularly if meningitis is suspected, infectious disease colleagues. Conservative treatment consists of strict bed rest and elevation of the head at least 30°. In addition, patients should be advised to refrain from coughing, sneezing, nose blowing, and straining or Valsalva maneuvers. Stool softeners are recommended, as well as antiemetics to avoid emesis or retching, antitussives to

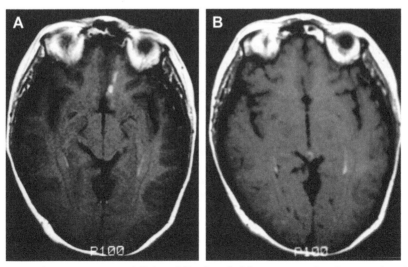

Fig. 3. Axial MRI scan post gadolinium following skull base trauma showing an enhancing lesion in the inferior-medial frontal lobe (*A*) with follow-up scan showing resolution of the lesion in 3 months (*B*).

avoid coughing, and strict blood pressure management. The goal of these measures is to reduce active flow through the leak, reduce CSF pressure, and allow healing of the defect to seal the leak, avoiding surgical intervention. In a series of 81 cases of traumatic CSF fistula, the overall rate of cessation with conservative treatment was 39.5% when used for 3 days. Resolution with conservative treatment of CSF fistulas involving temporal bone origin was 60%, whereas anterior skull base defects resolved 26.4% of the time with conservative treatment.[29] If conservative management is extended to 7 days, resolution rates improve to 85%, again with leaks of temporal bone origin healing with a significantly higher rate than those of anterior skull base origin.[30] The main reason for this discrepancy may be anatomic differences in the skull base bone and dural structures that are damaged with trauma to these subsites (ie, thin bone of the anterior skull base is more likely to cause significant dural lacerations than the thicker temporal bone).

Cerebrospinal Fluid Diversion

If there is persistence of the leak with conservative treatment, CSF diversion (most commonly with a lumber drain but occasionally serial lumbar punctures) is pursued. Lumbar drains are passive devices yet they require active management, as CSF cell count, protein and glucose measurements, and cultures should be collected frequently to monitor for meningitis, particularly if systemic signs exist. Average drainage rates are around 10 mL per hour. Optimal drainage lowers CSF pressure to decompress the leak; however, if drainage is too high severe headaches and pneumocephalus may result from drawing of air through the skull base defect into the cranial vault. There is also the added risk of meningitis. The benefits are that the addition of CSF diversion to conservative measures raises success rates to 70% to 90% with the average duration of drainage being 6.5 days.[30,31] Another benefit of this treatment is that it can be performed at the bedside, even if patients are not stable enough to go to the operating room. Lumbar drains can also be used as an adjunctive treatment to increase the success rates following a variety of surgical repairs.[31]

SURGICAL MANAGEMENT
Transcranial Approach

Although CSF rhinorrhea was initially described in the seventeenth century, it was not until 1926 that Dandy[32] reported the first successful repair by using a bifrontal craniotomy for access and a fascia lata graft for repair. With this approach, access to the cribriform plate region and roof of the ethmoid is obtained via a frontal craniotomy. An extended craniotomy and skull base dissection are required to access defects in the sphenoid sinus. After craniotomy the brain is retracted and the site of the defect is identified. Multiple tissues can be used for repair including fascia lata grafts, muscle plugs, and pedicled galeal or pericranial flaps. Tissue sealants, such as fibrin glue, can be used to hold the graft in position; however, this will only last a few weeks, leading the authors to prefer suture closure to the dura distal to the defect, which more securely holds the graft in place. Reported success rates vary; however, recurrence rates as high as 27% have been reported.[33] The clear advantage of this approach is that it provides direct access to the defect and allows for repair of multiple sites; however, with high reported failure rates, the morbidity of a craniotomy, and brain retraction (including potential hematoma, seizures, and anosmia), extracranial techniques are now preferred in most circumstances. At present these techniques are mostly used in patients who require a craniotomy and exposure of the skull base to treat associated intracranial pathology.

Extracranial Approach

The first extracranial approach was described by Dohlman[34] in 1948, when he used a naso-orbital incision to repair a CSF leak. Dissection is then carried into the sinus cavities through the external incision for trans-sinus access to the skull base defect. The defect is identified and repaired directly using tissue grafts. Success rates with this approach range from 86% to 97%.[35,36] The benefits of this approach include improved success rates with decreased morbidity, including avoiding anosmia and brain retraction with improved exposure of the posterior wall of the frontal sinus, fovea ethmoidalis, cribriform plate, posterior ethmoids, sphenoid, and parasellar regions. Drawbacks include the necessity of a facial scar, facial numbness, orbital injury, and relative difficulty of dissection. Further intracranial pathology as well as leaks originating from the lateral aspects of the frontal and sphenoid sinuses cannot be addressed.

Transnasal Approach

Further advancements were made in 1952, when Hirsch[37] reported the successful closure of two sphenoid sinus CSF leaks via a transnasal approach. In 1964, Vrabec and Hallberg[38] repaired a cribriform defect using this approach. In an attempt to improve visualization, Lehrer and Deutsch[39] used a microscope; however, access and visualization of the lateral and superior walls of the sphenoid sinus were limited. Inherent to this approach is the risk of facial numbness and septal perforation, and with the advent of endoscopic techniques this approach became rarely used.

Endoscopic Endonasal Approach

Endoscopic techniques have emerged as the preferred approach to the repair of skull base defects since their initial description by Wigand[40] in 1981. This initial report described repair of a defect encountered during sinus surgery. In 1989 the first report of the use of rigid transnasal endoscopy for the endonasal repair of CSF rhinorrhea was described,[41] followed by a series of cases presented by Mattox and Kennedy[42] addressing CSF rhinorrhea with the aid of endoscopic visualization. Following identification and localization of the skull base defect, standard endoscopic techniques are used to expose the defect site. This approach provides excellent exposure of the ethmoid roof, cribriform plate, and the sphenoid sinus.

When lateral exposure in the sphenoid is necessary, endoscopic dissection of the pterygomaxillary space can be performed. Exposure of the posterior aspect of the frontal sinus may require an osteoplastic flap or simple trephine. If needed, intrathecal fluorescein can be used to aid in identification of the skull base defect. Associated meningoencephaloceles are then addressed with bipolar electrocautery.

Mucosa that is adherent to dura must be dissected away. It is critical that the mucosa surrounding the skull base defect be removed for approximately half a centimeter. This technique both stimulates osteogenesis (thickening the bone surrounding the defect) and improves graft incorporation. Following site preparation, the decision for graft type can be made.

The choice of graft material has been a source of debate for some time; however, based on a recent meta-analysis it appears graft material does not affect success rate as long as sound surgical technique is used.[43] Graft choices include temporalis fascia, fascia lata, muscle plugs, mucosal grafts (with or without bone), autogenous fat, free cartilage grafts (from the nasal septum or auricle), and free bone grafts (from the nasal septum, calvarium, or iliac crest). For small defects, free mucosal or free fascial grafts can be placed in an overlay fashion. Significant overcorrection should be performed when forming the graft, as one can expect approximately 20% shrinkage in free mucosal graft size, starting in the first few postoperative days. Large defects at risk for secondary encephalocele are sometimes treated by placement of a bone or cartilaginous graft in an underlay fashion, with a fascial or mucosal graft placed as an overlay to form a watertight seal. In the authors' experience, this is usually not necessary. For large skull base defects the use of vascularized pedicled mucosal flaps are preferred, and this method is discussed in the following section.

In general, the authors' technique involves the placement of an inlay dural substitute graft (ie, Duragen; Integra, Plainsboro, NJ, USA) followed by a mucosal graft in the case of small defects or a vascularized pedicle flap for larger defects. Following graft placement, a sealant (such as fibrin glue) can be used to hold the graft in place. Absorbable nasal packing (gel-foam) is usually placed directly against the mucosal surface of the graft for additional support, followed by placement of nonabsorbable packing for further support and hemostasis. Packs are usually removed in 5 to 7 days, and antistaphylococcal antibiotic coverage should be used while nonabsorbable packs are in place.

Postoperatively the patient should be placed on conservative measures (as previously discussed). As dissection occurs through a contaminated operative field, most surgeons elect to use perioperative antibiotics. Antibiotic choice should have good CSF penetration (eg, ceftriaxone). At a minimum an antistaphylococcal antibiotic should be given postoperatively if nonabsorbable nasal packing is used. Admission to the intensive care unit for monitoring and frequent neurologic status checks should be considered for the first 24 hours to monitor for complications such as hematoma or cerebral edema, although this is institution dependent. If a lumbar drain is in place from prior attempts to slow CSF drainage, or if one was placed intraoperatively, it should be actively managed as discussed previously. Following removal of the nasal packing, serial nasal endoscopies should be performed for debridement of any crusting and to inspect the operative site. Care should be taken not to disrupt the graft during debridements, and patients should avoid strenuous activity or straining for approximately 6 weeks following the repair.

The endonasal endoscopic technique offers several advantages, including excellent visualization and identification of the defect as well as graft placement. Reported outcomes are excellent, with success rates of 90% for primary procedures and 96% for secondary endoscopic repair. The approach is remarkably well tolerated and complication rates are low, but present the risk for hemorrhage, infection, and graft failure.

Surgical Defects

CSF leaks after FESS tend to be small in size, less than 5 mm, and amenable to closure using any combination of inlaid bone, overlaid fascia, or free mucosal graft. However, over the past few years advances in endonasal endoscopic tumor removals have resulted in larger dural defects and have necessitated development of newer vascularized techniques to reconstruct the skull base. Although devascularized, layered reconstruction techniques of large skull base defects have been extensively described; they often result in high incidence of CSF leak and risk of meningitis. The use of vascularized mucosal pedicled flaps has been the most significant advancement in skull base reconstruction over the past decade.[44–46] The use of the posteriorly based pedicled nasal septal flap has become the primary mode of reconstruction following extensive endoscopic cranial base resections,[47] and decreased CSF leak rates following extensive endoscopic skull base reconstruction have been documented.[45] This flap is raised endoscopically (**Fig. 4**) and is based on the posterior septal artery (**Fig. 5**). Correct harvesting of this flap allows rotation of the flap in the

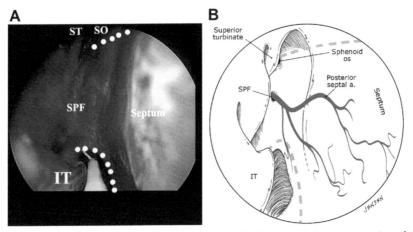

Fig. 4. Endoscopic view of the posterior nasal cavity (*A*) with an artist's representation of the same view (*B*). Dashed lines mark the location of cuts for the posteriorly based nasal septal flap. IT, inferior turbinate; SO, sphenoid os; SPF, sphenopalatine fossa; ST, superior turbinate.

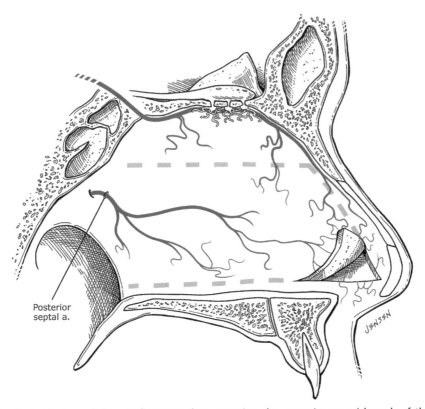

Fig. 5. Axial view of the nasal septum demonstrating the posterior septal branch of the sphenopalatine artery.

posterior, superior, inferior, or lateral directions. This flap is large enough to cover maximal dural defects extending from the frontal sinus to sella and from orbit to orbit (ie, craniofacial resection defect).[45] This flap can be used successfully in pediatric patients older than 14 years, but caution is recommended in younger patients, and it may not be a viable option in patients younger than 10 years, due to inadequate length.[48] Following endoscopic skull base reconstruction, it is often difficult to assess the integrity of the repair. Vascularized flaps have a characteristic appearance (mucosal enhancement) on MRI, which can cause some confusion following tumor resection, as radiologists and surgeons unfamiliar with this appearance may confuse the flap with residual tumor because traditional graft material (fat, explanted muscle, and synthetics) do not enhance. However, its appearance to the trained eye makes it ideal for monitoring the integrity of the skull base repair.[49] When a nasoseptal flap cannot be used, an anteriorly based pericranial flap can be elevated using minimally invasive techniques and placed intranasally without a craniotomy.[50] Other vascularized flaps available for endonasal skull base reconstruction include middle and inferior turbinate pedicled flaps,[51–53] temporoparietal fascia flap,[54] and palatal flap.[55]

CLINICAL QUESTIONS
Do Prophylactic Antibiotics Prevent Meningitis in Posttraumatic CSF Leaks?

Bacterial meningitis is the major cause of morbidity and mortality in patients with CSF leaks, making antibiotic prophylaxis a reasonable suggestion; however, this topic has been the source of significant controversy. The primary concern is that a CSF leak presents a direct route of infection from the contaminated nasal cavity to the intracranial space; however, unwarranted antibiotic use has the potential to select for resistant organisms. The reported incidence of meningitis in patients with posttraumatic CSF fistulas varies widely from 2% to 50%, with 10% being a generally accepted rate.[56–59]

Most of the controversy stems from two separate meta-analyses published 1 year apart. In 1997 Brodie[58] published a meta-analysis that showed a statistically significant reduction in the incidence of meningitis with prophylactic antibiotic therapy for patients with traumatic CSF leakage. This article was followed by a meta-analysis published in 1998 by Villalobos and colleagues,[60] which concluded that antibiotic prophylaxis after basilar skull fracture does not decrease the incidence of meningitis, independent of active CSF leak. However, critiques of these meta-analyses point out that neither of these studies included an extensive review of the literature and that the conclusions drawn were based mainly on retrospective and observational studies.[61] Further, it was suggested that the meta-analysis by Brodie omitted one of the largest case series addressing this question.[62] Recently a Cochrane Database review was performed to address these deficiencies. The analysis included 208 patients from 4 randomized controlled trials and an additional 2168 patients from 17 nonrandomized controlled trials. The analysis concluded that the evidence does not support the use of prophylactic antibiotics to reduce the risk of meningitis in patients with basilar skull fractures or basilar skull fractures with active CSF leak.[61] Analysis of both randomized and nonrandomized controlled trials failed to show a benefit or adverse effects of prophylactic antibiotic use in patients with active CSF leak; therefore, the current available literature suggests that prophylactic antibiotics do not decrease the risk of meningitis. It should be stated that perioperative antibiotics are indicated for surgical repair of CSF leaks, and in certain circumstances (such as active bacterial rhinosinusitis or grossly contaminated tract leading to the intracranial cavity) antibiotic coverage is reasonable.

Strength of evidence: Grade A

Does Early Surgical Repair Prevent Meningitis in Patients with Traumatic CSF Leaks?

Multiple factors seem to affect the rate of meningitis, including the duration of CSF leakage, the site of the skull base defect, and active sinus infections. Patients with traumatic CSF leaks lasting more than 7 days have been shown to have an estimated eightfold to tenfold increase in the risk of meningitis.[56,57] This finding has led some investigators to advocate surgical repair of CSF leaks that are persistent after 7 days of conservative treatment.[6] However, in some series conservative treatment has been associated with a high incidence of meningitis.[63] Furthermore, it has been shown that endoscopic closure of defects prevented meningitis in patients with and without a history of CSF infection.[64] These data lead the authors and many investigators to recommend early (less than 7 days) or urgent (less than 3 days) closure of traumatic CSF leaks as long as the patient is a suitable candidate for endoscopic closure.[6,63,64] However, in these studies it is difficult to assess the long-term risk of meningitis following surgical repair, as delayed cases of meningitis have been reported. Harvey and colleagues[65] looked to address this long-term risk and found that surgical repair results in decreased incidence of intracranial complications (including meningitis) over the long term. After assessment of risk factors for development of complications, they concluded that in patients with small nonleaking encephaloceles without adjacent infection, early surgical repair may not be indicated.

Strength of evidence: Grade C

SUMMARY

Indications for surgical intervention on traumatic CSF leaks include failure of conservative measures, identification of a CSF leak during FESS or skull base surgery, large skull base defects unlikely to heal with conservative measures (particularly if associated with pneumocephalus), or indication for associated surgical procedure to address other intracranial pathology. Recognizing that a single management strategy cannot possibly direct the care of each patient, given the varied mechanism of injury and patient presentations; the authors suggest the following evaluations to guide management.

Nonsurgical Trauma

When a patient presents with a nonsurgical traumatic CSF leak, fluid should be sent immediately for β_2-transferrin testing (as in some institutions this is a send-out test and may take several days to receive the result). If positive, conservative measures should be rapidly initiated and a high-resolution CT scan should be obtained for localization of the skull base defect. If needed, an MRI scan or cisternograms may be obtained for additional information/confirmation as already discussed. If the defect is in the anterior skull base, conservative treatment should be performed for 3 days. At this point, if the leak persists consideration of CSF diversion or endoscopic repair should be discussed in a multidisciplinary fashion. If CSF diversion is initiated and the leak is persistent, definitive repair (preferably endoscopic) should be performed around CSF leak day 7. If the CSF leak originates in the temporal bone, conservative measures should be continued for 5 to 7 days followed by CSF diversion for an additional 7 days, as these are more likely to close spontaneously and less likely to result in meningitis. Further operative repair of these defects cannot be addressed endoscopically, and definitive surgical repair of these defects can carry significant morbidity. If the leak persists for 2 weeks, definitive surgical repair should be performed.

Special consideration should be given to patients with coexistent intracranial pathology. If significant brain edema is present, early repair is likely to fail in the setting of elevated intracranial pressure. However, if the patient requires neurosurgical intervention, it is reasonable to repair coexistent CSF leaks at the same time. If a significant defect exists early definitive repair should be initiated, as conservative therapies are likely to fail. Perioperative antibiotics should be administered for surgical repair. If the patient is too ill to tolerate surgical repair, conservative measures should be continued until the patient is stable enough to undergo an operation.

Surgical Trauma

Intraoperative CSF leaks recognized at the time of surgery (either FESS or skull base procedures) should be immediately repaired. For planned dural resections, reconstruction should be "watertight." If recognition is delayed by days, weeks, or months, it is reasonable, although not the authors' practice, to initiate a short period of conservative therapy (a few days to 1 week). The leak should be confirmed and identified (as already discussed), and repaired if the leak persists for 1 week despite conservative measures. One should recognize that the later the CSF leak presents following the procedure, the less likely it is to resolve with conservative measures alone. Moreover, if the leak is massive in nature, early surgical intervention is indicated.

Traumatic CSF leaks are infrequent complications of craniomaxillofacial trauma or sinus/skull base surgery, but carry significant morbidity and mortality if not promptly recognized and appropriately managed. The main complication of CSF leaks is meningitis; however, tension pneumocephalus, meningoencephaloceles, and brain abscesses do occur. Identification and localization are critical to management. Conservative therapies should be initiated immediately, and consideration for operative intervention should involve a multidisciplinary team consisting of otolaryngology, neurosurgery, trauma, craniomaxillofacial surgery and, if meningitis is suspected, infectious disease physicians. The current evidence fails to show any benefit or adverse effects of prophylactic antibiotics, and it appears that endoscopic closure of persistent CSF leaks can prevent meningitis. This procedure has a high success rate in both primary and secondary surgery, and should be the primary approach for repair of posttraumatic anterior skull base CSF leaks.

EBM Question	Author's reply
Does spontaneous CSF leaks represent a distinct clinical entity and a variant of idiopathic intracranial hypertension?	Spontaneous CSF are both associated with raised ICP and idiopathic intracranial hypertension
Does a reduction in CSF pressure alone lead to resolution of CSF leaks?	Case reports describe resolution of CSF leaks with both diversion and other methods of CSF pressure reduction.
Does decreasing ICP, transiently or long-term, improve outcomes of endoscopic closure of spontaneous CSF leaks?	CSF pressure modifying medications and diversion have been shown to improve the longterm morbidity of IIH patients.

REFERENCES

1. Han CY, Backous DD. Basic principles of cerebrospinal fluid metabolism and intracranial pressure homeostasis. Otolaryngol Clin North Am 2005;38:569–76.
2. Har-El G. What is "spontaneous" cerebrospinal fluid rhinorrhea? Classification of cerebrospinal fluid leaks. Ann Otol Rhinol Laryngol 1999;108:323–6.

3. Loew F, Pertuiset B, Chaumier EE, et al. Traumatic, spontaneous and postoperative CSF rhinorrhea. Adv Tech Stand Neurosurg 1984;11:169–207.
4. Kerman M, Cirak B, Dagtekin A. Management of skull base fractures. Neurosurg Q 2002;12:23–41.
5. Friedman JA, Ebersold MJ, Quast LM. Post-traumatic cerebrospinal fluid leakage. World J Surg 2001;25:1062–6.
6. Banks CA, Palmer JN, Chiu AG, et al. Endoscopic closure of CSF rhinorrhea: 193 cases over 21 years. Otolaryngol Head Neck Surg 2009;140:826–33.
7. Kerr JT, Chu FW, Bayles SW. Cerebrospinal fluid rhinorrhea: diagnosis and management. Otolaryngol Clin North Am 2005;38:597–611.
8. Schlosser RJ, Wilensky EM, Grady MS, et al. Elevated intracranial pressures in spontaneous cerebrospinal fluid leaks. Am J Rhinol 2003;17:191–5.
9. Badia L, Loughran S, Lund V. Primary spontaneous cerebrospinal fluid rhinorrhea and obesity. Am J Rhinol 2001;15:117–9.
10. Schlosser RJ, Bolger WE. Significance of empty sella in cerebrospinal fluid leaks. Otolaryngol Head Neck Surg 2003;128:32–8.
11. Fain J, Chabannes J, Peri G, et al. [Frontobasal injuries and CSF fistulas. Attempt at an anatomoclinical classification. Therapeutic incidence]. Neurochirurgie 1975;21(6):493–506 [in French].
12. Kirsch AP. Diagnosis of cerebrospinal fluid rhinorrhea: lack of specificity of the glucose oxidase test tape. J Pediatr 1967;71:718–9.
13. Katz RT, Kaplan PE. Glucose oxidase sticks and cerebrospinal fluid rhinorrhea. Arch Phys Med Rehabil 1985;66:391–3.
14. Meurman OH, Irjala K, Suonpaa J, et al. A new method for the identification of cerebrospinal fluid leakage. Acta Otolaryngol 1979;87:366–9.
15. Oberascher G, Arrer E. Efficiency of various methods of identifying cerebrospinal fluid in oto- and rhinorrhea. ORL J Otorhinolaryngol Relat Spec 1986;48:320–5.
16. Normansell DE, Stacy EK, Booker CF, et al. Detection of beta-2 transferrin in otorrhea and rhinorrhea in a routine clinical laboratory setting. Clin Diagn Lab Immunol 1994;1:68–70.
17. Tripathi RC, Morrison N, Gulbarnson R, et al. Tau fraction of transferrin is present in human aqueous humor and is not unique to cerebrospinal fluid. Exp Eye Res 1990;50:541–7.
18. Storey EL, Anderson GJ, Mack U, et al. Desialylated transferrin as a serological marker of chronic alcohol ingestion. Lancet 1987;1(8545):1292–4.
19. Arrer E, Meco C, Oberascher G, et al. Beta-trace protein as a marker for cerebrospinal fluid rhinorrhea. Clin Chem 2002;48:939–41.
20. Meco C, Oberascher G, Arrer E, et al. Beta-trace protein test: new guidelines for the reliable diagnosis of cerebrospinal fluid fistula. Otolaryngol Head Neck Surg 2003;129:508–17.
21. Lloyd MN, Kimber PM, Burrows EH. Post-traumatic cerebrospinal fluid rhinorrhoea: modern high-definition computed tomography is all that is required for the effective demonstration of the site of leakage. Clin Radiol 1994;49(2):100–3.
22. Messerklinger W. Nasal endoscopy: demonstration, localization and differential diagnosis of nasal liquorrhea. HNO 1972;20:268–70 [in German].
23. Keerl R, Weber RK, Draf W, et al. Use of sodium fluorescein solution for detection of cerebrospinal fluid fistulas: an analysis of 420 administrations and reported complications in Europe and the United States. Laryngoscope 2004;114:266–72.
24. Stone JA, Castillo M, Neelon B, et al. Evaluation of CSF leaks: high resolution CT compared with contrast enhanced CT and radionuclide cisternography. AJNR Am J Neuroradiol 1999;20:706–12.

25. Curnes JT, Vincent LM, Kowalsky RJ, et al. CSF rhinorrhea: detection and localization using overpressure cisternography with Tc-99m-DTPA. Radiology 1985;154:795–9.
26. Sillers MJ, Morgan E, El Gammal T. Magnetic resonance cisternography and thin coronal computerized tomography in the evaluation of cerebrospinal fluid rhinorrhea. Am J Rhinol 1997;11:387–92.
27. Zapalac JS, Marple BF, Schwade ND. Skull base cerebrospinal fluid fistulas: a comprehensive diagnostic algorithm. Otolaryngol Head Neck Surg 2002;126:669–76.
28. Mostafa BE, Khafaqi A. Combined HRCT and MRI in the detection of CSF rhinorrhea. Skull Base 2004;14:157–62.
29. Yilmazlar S, Arslan E, Kocaeli H, et al. Cerebrospinal fluid leakage complicating skull base fractures: analysis of 81 cases. Neurosurg Rev 2006;29:64–71.
30. Bell RB, Dierks EJ, Homer L, et al. Management of cerebrospinal fluid leak associated with craniomaxillofacial trauma. J Oral Maxillofac Surg 2004;62(6):676–84.
31. Shapiro SA, Scully T. Closed continuous drainage of cerebrospinal fluid via a lumbar subarachnoid catheter for treatment of prevention of cranial/spinal cerebrospinal fluid fistula. Neurosurgery 1992;30(2):241–5.
32. Dandy WE. Pneumocephalus (intracranial pneumocele or aerocele). Arch Surg 1926;12:949–82.
33. Ray BS, Bergland RM. Cerebrospinal fluid fistula: clinical aspects, techniques of localization and methods of closure. J Neurosurg 1967;30:399–405.
34. Dohlman G. Spontaneous cerebrospinal fluid rhinorrhea. Acta Otolaryngol Suppl (Stockh) 1948;67:20–3.
35. McCormack B, Cooper PR, Persky M, et al. Extracranial repair of cerebrospinal fluid fistulas: technique and results in 37 patients. Neurosurgery 1990;27:412–7.
36. Persky MS, Rothstein SG, Breda SD, et al. Extracranial repair of cerebrospinal fluid otorhinorrhea. Laryngoscope 1991;101:134–6.
37. Hirsch O. Successful closure of cerebrospinal fluid rhinorrhea by endonasal surgery. Arch Otolaryngol 1952;56:1–13.
38. Vrabec DP, Hallberg OE. Cerebrospinal fluid rhinorrhea. Arch Otolaryngol 1964;80:218–29.
39. Lehrer J, Deutsch H. Intranasal surgery for cerebrospinal fluid rhinorrhea. Mt Sinai J Med 1970;37:113–38.
40. Wigand ME. Transnasal ethmoidectomy under endoscopic control. Rhinology 1981;19:7–15.
41. Papay FA, Maggiano H, Dominquez S, et al. Rigid endoscopic repair of paranasal sinus cerebrospinal fluid fistulas. Laryngoscope 1989;99:1195–201.
42. Mattox DE, Kennedy DW. Endoscopic management of cerebrospinal fluid leaks and encephaloceles. Laryngoscope 1990;100:857–62.
43. Hegazy HM, Carrau RL, Snyderman CH, et al. Transnasal endoscopic repair of cerebrospinal fluid rhinorrhea: a meta-analysis. Laryngoscope 2000;110:1166–72.
44. Harvey RJ, Nogueira JF, Schlosser RJ, et al. Closure of large skull base defects after endoscopic transnasal craniotomy. J Neurosurg 2009;111(2):371–9.
45. Kassam AB, Thomas A, Carrau RL, et al. Endoscopic reconstruction of the cranial base using a pedicled nasoseptal flap. Neurosurgery 2008;63(1 Suppl 1):ONS44–52.
46. El-Sayed IH, Roediger FC, Goldberg AN, et al. Endoscopic reconstruction of skull base defects with the nasal septal flap. Skull Base 2008;18(6):385–94.
47. Hadad G, Bassagasteguy L, Carrau RL, et al. A novel reconstructive technique after endoscopic expanded endonasal approaches: vascular pedicle nasoseptal flap. Laryngoscope 2006;116:1882–6.

48. Shah RN, Surowitz JB, Patel MR, et al. Endoscopic pedicled nasoseptal flap reconstruction for pediatric skull base defects. Laryngoscope 2009;119(6):1067–75.
49. Kang MD, Escott E, Thomas AJ, et al. The MR imaging appearance of the vascular pedicle nasoseptal flap. AJNR Am J Neuroradiol 2009;30(4):781–6.
50. Zanation AM, Snyderman CH, Carrau RL, et al. Minimally invasive endoscopic pericranial flap: a new method for endonasal skull base reconstruction. Laryngoscope 2009;119(1):13–8.
51. Harvey RJ, Sheahan PO, Schlosser RJ. Inferior turbinate pedicle flap for endoscopic skull base defect repair. Am J Rhinol Allergy 2009;23(5):522–6.
52. Prevedello DM, Barges-Coll J, Fernandez-Miranda JC, et al. Middle turbinate flap for skull base reconstruction: cadaveric feasibility study. Laryngoscope 2009; 119(11):2094–8.
53. Fortes FS, Carrau RL, Snyderman CH, et al. The posterior pedicle inferior turbinate flap: a new vascularized flap for skull base reconstruction. Laryngoscope 2007;117(8):1329–32.
54. Fortes FS, Carrau RL, Snyderman CH, et al. Transpterygoid transposition of a temporoparietal fascia flap: a new method for skull base reconstruction after endoscopic expanded endonasal approaches. Laryngoscope 2007;117(6):970–6.
55. Oliver CL, Hackman TG, Carrau RL, et al. Palatal flap modifications allow pedicled reconstruction of the skull base. Laryngoscope 2008;118(12):2102–6.
56. Leech PJ, Paterson A. Conservative and operative management for cerebrospinal-fluid leakage after closed head injury. Lancet 1973;1(7811):1013–6.
57. Mincy JE. Posttraumatic cerebrospinal fluid fistula of the frontal fossa. J Trauma 1966;6:618–22.
58. Brodie HA. Prophylactic antibiotics for posttraumatic cerebrospinal fluid fistulae: a meta-analysis. Arch Otolaryngol Head Neck Surg 1997;123:749–52.
59. MacGee EE, Cauthen JC, Brackett CE. Meningitis following acute traumatic cerebrospinal fluid fistula. J Neurosurg 1970;33:312–6.
60. Villalobos T, Arango C, Kubilis P, et al. Antibiotic prophylaxis after basilar skull fractures: a meta-analysis. Clin Infect Dis 1998;27:364–9.
61. Ratilal BO, Costa J, Sampaio C. Antibiotic prophylaxis for preventing meningitis in patients with basilar skull fractures. Cochrane Database Syst Rev 2006;(1): CD004884.
62. Daudia A, Biswas D, Jones NS. Risk of meningitis with cerebrospinal fluid rhinorrhea. Ann Otol Rhinol Laryngol 2007;116(12):902–5.
63. Bernal-Sprekelsen M, Bleda-Vázquez C, Carrau RL. Ascending meningitis secondary to traumatic cerebrospinal fluid leaks. Am J Rhinol 2000;14:257–9.
64. Bernal-Sprekelsen M, Alobid I, Mullol J, et al. Closure of cerebrospinal fluid leaks prevents ascending bacterial meningitis. Rhinology 2005;43:277–81.
65. Harvey RJ, Smith JE, Wise SK, et al. Intracranial complications before and after endoscopic skull base reconstruction. Am J Rhinol 2008;22:516–21.

Osteoma of the Skull Base and Sinuses

Christos Georgalas, PhD, DLO, FRCS(ORL-HNS)[a],*, John Goudakos, MD[b],
Wytske J. Fokkens, MD, PhD[c]

KEYWORDS

- Osteoma • Draf type 3 procedure • Endoscopic procedures
- Endoscopic modified lothrop

EBM Question	Level of Evidence	Grade of Recommendation
What are the limits of the endoscopic approach?	4	C

Osteoma is a benign, slow-growing bone tumor consisting primarily of well-differentiated mature, compact, or cancellous bone. Osteoma is the most common benign tumor of the paranasal sinuses with a point prevalence of 3%, as demonstrated in 2 computed tomography (CT) radiological studies of 1500[1] and 1889[2] patients respectively.

AGE AND SEX

Osteomas occur more often in men, with a variable male-to-female ratio of 1.3:1.0[1] to 1.5:1.0.[2,3] Their peak incidence is between the fourth and sixth decades, with an average age at presentation of 50 years.[1,2]

LOCATION

Most osteomas (58%[1] to 68%[3]) involve the frontal sinus (37% arise in the immediate vicinity of the nasofrontal duct and 21% above and lateral to the frontal ostium).[1] The

[a] Department of Otolaryngology, Endoscopic Skull Base Centre, Academic Medical Centre, Amsterdam, Meibergdreef 9, 1105 AZ, The Netherlands
[b] Department of Otolaryngology, AHEPA University Hospital, Aristotle University of Thessaloniki, Salonika, Thessaloniki, Greece
[c] Department of Otolaryngology, Academic Medical Centre, Amsterdam, Meibergdreef 9, 1105 AZ, The Netherlands
* Corresponding author.
E-mail address: cgeorgalas@amc.uva.nl

Otolaryngol Clin N Am 44 (2011) 875–890
doi:10.1016/j.otc.2011.06.008
0030-6665/11/$ – see front matter © 2011 Elsevier Inc. All rights reserved.

ethmoid sinus is the second most common area to be involved, whereas maxillary sinuses are affected in about 20% of cases, and sphenoid sinuses are rarely involved.[1] Osteomas can occur in conjunction with Gardner syndrome (familial adenomatous polyposis) **(Fig. 1)**, an autosomal dominant condition consisting of multiple osteomas, soft tissue tumors (including skin cysts and desmoid tumors), and colon polyps with a high propensity toward malignant transformation.[4] As osteomas tend to appear an average of 17 years before the colon polyps, early gastroenterology referral is strongly advised.[5]

ETIOLOGY OF OSTEOMA

There are 3 main pathogenetic theories regarding the etiology of osteomas: developmental, traumatic, and infective.[6,7] According to the developmental theory, as proposed by Cohnheim, osteomas arise from stem cells of the junctional area between the frontal and ethmoid bone. This is supported by the fact that osteomas frequently occur at the fontoethmoid suture line where the frontal sinus (membranous bone) borders the ethmoid labyrinth (endochondral ossification). However, this theory does not explain osteomas found in other locations. The traumatic theory, as proposed by Gerber, suggests that osteomas arise as an abnormal proliferative response to trauma and is supported by both the higher incidence of osteomas in men and the development of osteomas during puberty, when the rate of skeletal development is at its peak.[8] However, most osteomas are detected later in life and the great majority of patients do not report any history of trauma, whereas an increased incidence of osteomata in patients undergoing multiple endoscopic sinus surgery procedures has never been documented. Alternatively, it has been suggested that osteomas may arise as a result of infection stimulating osteoblasts within the mucoperiosteal lining of the sinus, which in turn may become secondarily calcified. Although there is an association between osteoma and sinusitis, the cause-and-effect relationship is not clear, and in up to 63% of cases, osteomas arise in healthy sinuses.[2] Other less substantiated theories suggest that osteomas may be osteodysplastic lesions, osteogenic hamartomas, embryonic bone rests, or the result of ossification of sinus polyps. However, none of these hypotheses have been proven.[4]

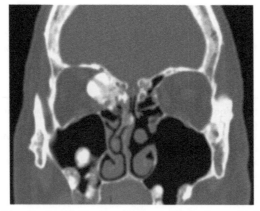

Fig. 1. A 51-year-old patient with Gardner syndrome. Note the multiple osteomata of the facial skeleton occurring in unusual locations, including the orbita, maxillary sinus, and zygomatic bone.

HISTOLOGY OF OSTEOMA

Macroscopically, osteomas are round or oval, hard, ivory-white, bosselated, well-circumscribed lesions attached to the underlying bone by a broad base or occasionally by a small stalk and covered by a thin layer of fibrous periosteum.[9] Histologically, osteomas can be classified into 3 types: ivory or compact, mature or cancellous, or spongiotic and mixed.[6,10] Ivory osteomas usually have a sessile base and are characterized by hard bone with a thick matrix containing only a small amount of fibrous tissue and minimal marrow. Cancellous osteomas often have a pedunculated base and are composed of cancellous bone with intertrabecular hematopoietic bone marrow or fat, whereas mixed osteomas share characteristics from both types (**Fig. 2**).[9,10]

GROWTH

In a study of 13 osteomas with serial radiographs, the average growth rate was 1.61 mm per year, ranging from 0.44 to 6.00 mm per year.[11] It has been shown that most osteomas recur infrequently even after incomplete removal.[12] However, given enough time, osteomas can recur,[13,14] and indeed accelerated regrowth following incomplete removal has been documented.[15] Malignant transformation of an osteoma has never been described, and osteomas should not be considered neoplastic lesions.[10]

CLINICAL CHARACTERISTICS OF OSTEOMA

Most osteomata are asymptomatic, slow-growing lesions diagnosed incidentally in imaging studies. Only 4%[1] to 10%[16] of all osteomas produce clinical symptoms, with osteomas of the frontoethmoidal region tending to be associated with earlier symptoms. Such symptoms are most commonly frontal pressure or headache,[17,18] either directly resulting from the lesion or indirectly from impaired drainage of the frontal sinus with or without concomitant chronic rhinosinusitis. The incidence of headache in various osteoma series varies between 52%[19] and 100% (**Table 1**).[17]

Complete obstruction of a sinus ostium by an osteoma may lead to secondary formation of mucocele.[25,26] When an osteoma extends beyond the confines of the sinuses, it may produce an external deformity (**Fig. 3**).[27] Orbital extension may lead to proptosis and periorbital pain, as well as chemosis and diplopia if the oculomotor muscles are affected[28–30] or epiphora if the nasolacrimal duct is compressed (**Fig. 4**)[31,32] and rarely

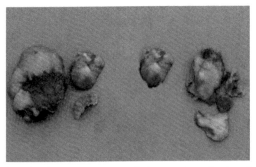

Fig. 2. Fragments of a mixed osteoma removed via an external osteoplastic flap approach. Note the thin mucosal layer overlying the osteoma.

Table 1
Osteomata case series

Study, Year, Journal	Cases	Presenting Symptoms	Location	Tumor Grade	Procedure	Outcome	Complications	Follow-Up (Months)
Brodish et al[20]	9	Headache	9 frontoethmoidal	nr	9 end	0	2 CSF leaks	40
Schick et al[17]	34	Headache	23 frontal sinus 11 ethmoid	nr	23 end 11 open	3 residuals (end)	0	1–32
Chiu et al[21]	9	Headache 88% Sinusitis 66%	9 frontal sinus	I: 1 II: 2 III: 4 IV: 2	3 end 5 combined 1 open	nr	0	7.4
Dubin and Kuhn[22]	12	Headache 100%	12 frontal sinus	I: 3 III: 8 IV: 1	8 end 4 combined	2 residuals (open) 1 residuals (end)	1 frontal stenosis (open)	19.2
Bignami et al[23]	26	Headache 63% Nasal obstr 38%	26 frontal sinus	nr	11 end 13 combined 2 open	0 recurrences	0	40
Castelnuovo et al[19]	48	Headache 52%	18 frontal sinus 13 frontoethmoid 9 ethmoid 8 other	nr	22 end 26 open	nr	0	53 (end) 35 (open)
Seiberling et al[18]	23	Headache 62.5% Sinusitis 56.5%	18 frontal sinus 5 frontal recess	I: 5 II: 4 III: 6 IV: 8	2 combined 21 end	4 residuals	1 frontal stenosis (end)	33
Ledderose et al[24]	24	Headache 83% Sinusitis 87%	7 frontal sinus 7 frontal recess	I: 3 II: 5 III: 10 IV: 6	12 combined 8 end 4 open	95% satisfied[a] 1 pain increase	1 bleeding (combined) 1 bleeding (open)	nr

Abbreviations: CSF, cerebrospinal fluid; nr, not recorded.
[a] SNOT 20 questionnaire.

decreased visual acuity in cases of optic nerve compression.[33,34] Intracranial extension of the lesion can lead to intracranial mucocele with meningitis, cerebral abscess,[35–37] or even tension pneumocephalus (**Fig. 5**).[38] In our experience, headache is the sole presenting symptom of osteomas in the vast majority of cases, whereas the slow growth of an osteoma usually precludes eye symptoms, even in cases of significant orbital extension, unless a concomitant mucocele is present.

IMAGING

Although osteomata can be seen in simple sinus radiographs, the imaging modality of choice is thin-slice CT. This allows the precise estimation of the size and the location of the osteoma, as well as concurrent sinus pathology. Osteomata appear as well-circumscribed masses of heterogeneous consistency on CT, with hyperostotic (high signal) and spongiotic (lower signal) components (**Fig. 6**). The lower signal components may be confused with associated mucoceles. In such patients, magnetic resonance imaging is useful to assess the extent of the tumor as well as the presence of complications (mucoceles, orbital or intracranial extension).

INDICATIONS

Although it is generally agreed that symptomatic osteomas (unless there are serious contraindications) should be surgically excised, management of asymptomatic osteomata is controversial. In the case of small, uncomplicated osteomata, watchful waiting with interval radiologic imaging is usually advised. Savić and Djerić[39] recommend surgical removal of enlarging frontal sinus osteomas, those extending beyond the

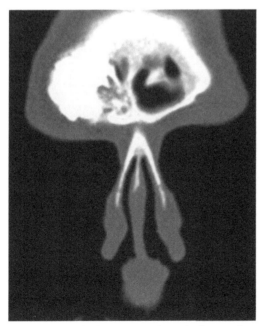

Fig. 3. Osteoma extending through the anterior frontal plate and associated with facial deformity.

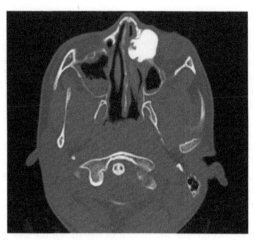

Fig. 4. A patient referred by the ophthalmologist where he attended with epiphora. Note the osteoma obstructing the nasolacrimal duct.

boundaries of the sinus, localized adjacent to the nasofrontal duct, associated with chronic sinusitis, or in patients complaining of headaches when all other causes have been excluded, as well as osteomas in the ethmoid sinuses, irrespective of their size. Smith and Calcaterra recommend surgery if the osteoma occupies more than 50% of the frontal sinus.[40] Our policy is to treat the following:

- Osteomas associated with symptoms (usually headache) after all other explanations for the symptoms have been excluded

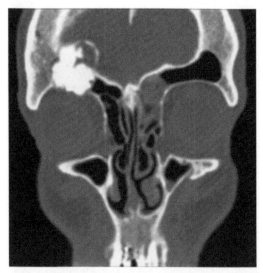

Fig. 5. Large osteoma of the frontal sinus in a patient presenting with headache. There was significant intracranial extension but the dura was intact and the patient had no neurologic complications.

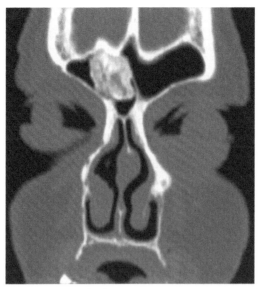

Fig. 6. Frontal sinus osteoma. Note the heterogeneous appearance on CT.

- Large (extending to more than 50% of the frontal sinus) or growing osteomas, as seen on serial CTs
- Osteomas associated with current (mucocele, orbital symptoms, neurologic symptoms, external deformity), imminent (complete obstruction of the frontal recess, intraorbital or intracranial extension) complications.

We do not operate small ethmoid osteomas, which, more often than not, are incidental CT findings with no clinical significance.

Lynch Procedure

One of the first methods used to treat symptomatic frontal or frontoethmoid osteomas was the external frontoethmoidectomy approach (Lynch procedure).[22] This has been used for small, medially or inferiorly situated tumors. However, it can lead to an unsightly scar, does not provide adequate access laterally, and has a high rate of frontal recess stenosis.[41]

Osteoplastic Flap Procedures

The osteoplastic approach, as popularized by Goodale and Montgomery,[42] has been the most widely used technique for frontal sinus osteomas. It provides excellent visualization and wide access to the frontal sinus, including its superior, posterior, and lateral aspects, although the nasofrontal duct and ethmoids may not always be adequately visualized. The osteoplastic flap procedure is well established, being in use for more than 40 years, and is technically accessible to most otolaryngologists. Nevertheless, it is an invasive procedure, with significant morbidity, including blood loss, impaired cosmesis, postoperative frontal pain, paresthesia, or anesthesia from supraorbital nerve damage and (rarely) in the case of intracranial entry, potentially devastating complications including cerebrospinal fluid (CSF) leak and meningitis. If the frontal sinus is obliterated, then the added morbidity of an abdominal incision for fat harvesting is introduced, as well as the risk of late mucocele formation, which can be as high as 9% after 2 years.[43]

Endoscopic Procedures

Endoscopic approaches to the nose and paranasal sinuses were introduced in the 1980s, and by the early 1990s the first cases of endoscopic management of ethmoid osteoma were published.[44,45] The accumulation of experience with endoscopic sinus surgery, technological advances, including the development of dedicated instruments (malleable forceps; 40-degree, 55-degree, and 70-degree curved diamond and cutting drills; straight high-speed neurosurgical drill; and dedicated bipolar intranasal diathermy forceps), improved endoscopes, and the introduction of CT navigation, expanded the limits of endoscopic approaches. On the other hand, the work of Draf, in systematizing the approaches to the frontal sinus,[46] laid the foundations of modern endoscopic frontal sinus surgery. Importantly, he described the type 3 ("Draf 3") procedure (endoscopic modified lothrop,[47] bilateral frontal sinus drillout,[48] median drainage procedure[49]) as a way to establish the widest possible transnasal access to the frontal sinus.

WHAT ARE THE LIMITS OF THE ENDOSCOPIC APPROACH?

As with most surgical techniques, Level 1 or 2 evidence is missing; however, Level 3 evidence can be collected using case series and retrospective cohorts. The evolution of these indications testifies to the progress affected in endoscopic surgery over the past decades.

Ethmoid Sinus

Endoscopic approaches to an ethmoid osteoma are relatively straightforward. The involvement of the cribriform plate is not a contraindication, as gentle drilling using a diamond burr until the osteoma is paper thin can help to remove the osteoma. Even extensive involvement of the orbit can usually be dealt with endoscopically; the limit being the anterior extension. Extension anteriorly to the nasolacrimal duct and under the skin usually requires a combined endoscopic/external (transconjuctival) approach in this case (see **Fig. 2**).

Frontal Sinus

Draf, in his seminal paper on the Fulda concept in 1991, suggested that any "large osteoma" was not amenable to an endoscopic approach and should be dealt with via an osteoplastic flap approach.[50]

Since then, 8 case series, including at least 5 osteomata each, have been published (see **Table 1**).

Brodish and colleagues[20] presented in 1999 a series of 8 osteomata treated endoscopically. They were removed with osteotomes and curettes and there were 2 incidences of (anticipated) CSF leaks. No specific indications were described for the endoscopic approach.

The first large series of sinonasal osteomata treated endoscopically was published by Schick and colleagues[17] in 2001. They suggested, on the basis of 35 patients, that exclusion criteria for an endoscopic approach included:

1. Intracranial extension
2. Large intraorbital involvement
3. Anteroposterior diameter of the frontal sinus smaller than 10 mm
4. Lateral extension over a virtual plane through the lamina papyracea
5. Erosion of the posterior or anterior wall of the frontal sinus.

However, the first systematic attempt to codify the limits of resection was by Chiu and colleagues in 2005.[21] Drawing from their experience with 9 osteomas between 1999 and 2003, they developed a grading system (**Table 2**) maintaining that only grades 1 and 2 osteomata can be removed endoscopically.

Essentially, their grading suggests that the 3 contraindications for endonasal removal of an osteoma are the following:

1. Base of attachment anteriorly or superiorly within the frontal sinus
2. Extension laterally to a virtual sagittal plane through the lamina papyracea
3. Complete obliteration of entire frontal sinus.

Castelnuovo and colleagues,[19] on the basis of 33 osteomata, suggested that an endoscopic approach was contraindicated in cases of:

1. Lateral extension to the sagittal plane passing through the lamina papyracea
2. Intracranial extension
3. Involvement of the posterior and anterior wall of the frontal sinus
4. Anteroposterior frontal sinus diameter smaller than 1 cm.

In 2007, Bignami and colleagues,[23] on the basis of 25 osteomata, supported Chiu and colleagues grading system and criteria for endoscopic removal. They stated that an endoscopic approach was not feasible in cases with:

1. Intracranial extension
2. Large orbital involvement
3. Anteroposterior diameter of the frontal sinus smaller than 10 mm
4. Lateral extension behind a virtual plane through the lamina papyracea
5. Erosion of the posterior or anterior wall of the frontal sinus.

Endoscopic surgery has been evolving at a very fast pace and a number of surgeons have challenged these assumptions. Just a year after the publication of the Chiu and colleagues classification, Dubin and Kuhn[22] published their results of successful endoscopic removal of 5 grade III tumors attached either superior-anteriorly in the frontal sinus or extending lateral to the plane of lamina papyracea. In this article, an osteoplastic flap was recommended only for removal of tumors with more than 2 cm of vertical extension into the frontal sinus or occupancy of 100% of the frontal sinus.

Table 2 Frontal sinus osteoma grading system	
Grade I	Base of attachment is posterior–inferior along the frontal recess. Tumor is medial to a virtual sagittal plane through the lamina papyracea. Anterior–posterior diameter of the lesion is *less* than 75% of the anterior–posterior dimension of the frontal recess.
Grade II	Base of attachment is posterior–inferior along the frontal recess. Tumor is medial to a virtual sagittal plane through the lamina papyracea. Anterior–posterior diameter of the lesion is *greater* than 75% of the anterior–posterior dimension of the frontal recess.
Grade III	Base of attachment is anterior or superiorly located within the frontal sinus AND/OR tumor extends lateral to a virtual sagittal plane through the lamina papyracea.
Grade IV	Tumor fills the entire frontal sinus

Data from Chiu AG, Schipor I, Cohen NA, et al. Surgical decisions in the management of frontal sinus osteomas. Am J Rhinol 2005;19(2):191–7.

In 2009, Seiberling and colleagues[18] reported their results of 23 patients with varying sizes of frontal sinus osteomas treated endoscopically, which included 8 patients with a grade IV tumor and 6 patients with a grade III tumor. A Draf 3 procedure was used for 15 of these tumors (including all grade III and IV tumors). In 4 of 8 grade IV (filling the entire frontal sinus) tumors, a residual was left toward the posterior frontal plate, as it was felt that the risk of penetrating the dura was too high. In 2 cases, a second procedure was necessary for the complete removal of the tumor, whereas in one patient with extensive orbital extension, an external blepharoplasty incision was used and an extended trephine incision was used in another patient.

In 2010, Ledderose and colleagues[24] proposed that, in carefully selected individual cases, it is possible to remove grade III and even grade IV osteomas endonasally. They described the endoscopic removal of 8 osteomas, 3 of which would have been classified as nonresectable endoscopically according to the Chiu and colleagues classification: specifically, 2 grade III tumors were removed via a Draf 2b approach and a grade IV tumor was removed via a Draf 3 approach.

What we know now is that, although there is no number of external approaches that can prove the limits of endoscopic surgery, a small number of endoscopic approaches (replicated in more than one center) can shatter the myth of "unresectability." We believe that it is not the anteroposterior diameter or the lateral extension of the osteoma that defines its resectability endoscopically, but rather the relation between the interorbital distance, the anteroposterior diameter of the frontal beak, and the lateral height of the frontal sinus. We have attempted to codify our experience with the endoscopic approach to osteomata as follows (Grade C recommendations):

1. Lateral extent
2. Large tumors attached to the posterior/superior frontal walls/more than 2 cm superiorly in the frontal sinus
3. Orbital extension
4. Intracranial extension
5. Anterior extension.

Lateral extent
Using the wide access provided by a Draf 3 procedure and curved drills, it is possible to access the lateral supraorbital ridge well beyond the medial orbit. We maintain that it is not the plane of lamina papyracea or the 2 cm lateral to it that define the lateral

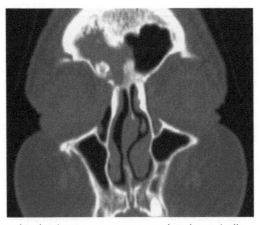

Fig. 7. Osteoma lateral to lamina papyracea removed endoscopically.

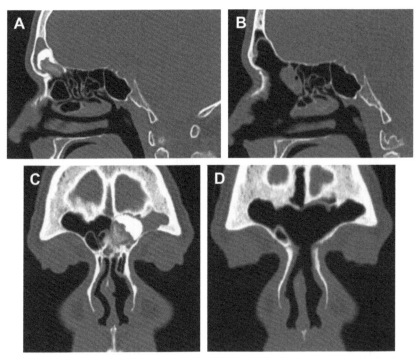

Fig. 8. (*A–D*) Preoperative and postoperative CT scans of a large osteoma attached to the posterior frontal sinus wall, extending more than 2 cm superiorly and completely obstructing the frontal sinus removed endoscopically.

limits of respectability, but rather the ratio of lateral tumor extension to *interorbital distance.* Following the removal of the superior septum and the drilling of the nasal beak, lateral access to the frontal sinus is restricted primarily by the orbital walls. In patients with relatively large intercanthal distance, the lateral access that can be

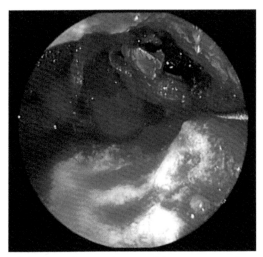

Fig. 9. Thinning out of the posterior attachment of the osteoma and removal with a curette: view through a Draf 3 procedure.

Table 3
Evolution of contraindications of endoscopic approach

Anatomic Limitations	Schick[17]	Chiu[21]	Dubin[22]	Bignami[23]	Castelnuovo[19]	Seiberling[18]	Ledderose[24]	AMC
Attachment anterior frontal plate	YES				YES			YES (when associated with large defect or very high attachment)
Attachment posterior frontal plate					YES	NO (may need to leave remnant)		NO
Attachment superior frontal sinus		YES				NO	NO	NO
Less than 1 cm frontal sinus diameter	YES			YES	YES			Relative
Extension more than 2 cm superiorly in frontal sinus			YES			NO	NO	NO
Lateral to lamina papyracea sagittal plane	YES			YES	YES	NO	NO	NO
2 cm lateral to orbit						NO	NO	NO
Erosion of anterior table	YES			YES	YES		YES	YES
Complete obstruction of frontal recess			YES			NO	NO	NO
Complete opacification of frontal sinus		YES				NO		NO
Intracranial extension/erosion of posterior table	YES			YES	YES			NO
Extension anterior to nasolacrimal duct								YES
(Significant) orbital extension	YES			YES		NO (may require additional incision)		NO

Abbreviation: AMC, Academic Medical Centre.

gained is increased, whereas the opposite is true for narrow nasal inlet (**Fig. 7**). Lateral access to the floor of the frontal sinus (orbital roof) may, however, be limited, as a recent study[51] confirmed.

Large tumors attached to the posterior/superior frontal walls/more than 2 cm superiorly in the frontal sinus
Similarly, tumors extending superiorly, to the posterior frontal plate, or associated with complete opacification of the frontal sinus can also be removed endoscopically (**Figs. 8** and **9**).

In many cases, we saw that the approach of such tumors was time consuming, as the curved drills operating at 10,000 rpm (as opposed to the 80,000-rpm straight drills) would frequently fail and had to be changed. In one such case, our approach was staged, and the osteoma was removed completely in the second approach, and with the use of a (much more effective) 80,000-rpm straight drill. The development in the future of high-speed curved drills may further facilitate the removal of such large laterally located osteomas.

Orbital extension
Orbital extension is not in itself a contraindication for an endonasal approach (see **Fig. 4**). However, as stated by others,[18] additional incisions may be required if the tumor extends *anteriorly*. We found that anterior extension (anteriorly to the nasolacrimal duct), rather than in the orbit per se, is an indication for an external incision. In most cases, the external approach can be performed via a subconjunctival incision, with no cosmetic consequences.

Intracranial extension
We maintain that limited endocranial extension does not always preclude the use of the endoscope. As we progress to manage intracranial/intradural tumors endoscopically, the limitation of posterior wall erosion/endocranial extension sounds irrelevant, with the proviso that the removal is done in combination with a endoscopically trained neurosurgeon.

Anterior extension
The one limitation to endonasal approaches that seems to withstand the test of time is anterior extension. Extension of the tumor through the anterior frontal plate is usually physically impossible to access endoscopically, whereas the associated bony defect and deformity necessitates an external approach for reconstruction (see **Fig. 3**).

The evolution of contraindications for the endoscopic approach is presented in **Table 3**.

SUMMARY

Advantages of the endoscopic approach include better close-up and 3-dimensional visualization of anatomic structures, absence of scars, smaller traumatic impact along the approach path, reduction of postoperative morbidity, preservation of the physiologic mucociliary drainage, less bleeding, and a shorter hospital stay. However, the endoscopic approach can make the management of potential intraoperative complications (massive bleeding, intracranial complications, CSF leak) more difficult and requires significant time commitment (for large osteomata, significantly more than an external approach) and highly sophisticated surgical tools.

We do not believe that the endonasal removal of osteomas is a procedure that should be undertaken lightly. Significant experience in all frontal sinus approaches, including Draf type 3 sinusotomy, is required, together with great facility in the use of the drill endonasally. Although temporal bone drilling is part of the curriculum in most residency programs, the development of similar skills for drilling in the anterior skull base is not required and is rarely acquired during training. As endoscopic sinus surgery comes of age, we expect that the skills required will be more widely shared. A new generation of surgeons will be moving forward the frontiers of endoscopic surgery, and we expect that what today are the "frontiers" of endonasal surgery will be standard procedures tomorrow.

EBM Question	Author's reply
What are the limits of the endoscopic approach?	1. Lateral extent – access on the orbital roof beyond midline a limitation 2. Large tumors attached to the posterior/superior frontal walls/more than 2 cm supe-riorly in the frontal sinus – relative limitation as very time consuming via endonasal approach 3. Orbital extension – not a limitation 4. Intracranial extension – not a limitation 5. Anterior extension – tumors with anterior table erosion and anterior to the nasolacrimal duct a limitation

REFERENCES

1. Earwaker J. Paranasal sinus osteomas: a review of 46 cases. Skeletal Radiol 1993;22(6):417–23.
2. Erdogan N, Demir U, Songu M, et al. A prospective study of paranasal sinus osteomas in 1,889 cases: changing patterns of localization. Laryngoscope 2009; 119(12):2355–9.
3. McHugh JB, Mukherji SK, Lucas DR. Sino-orbital osteoma: a clinicopathologic study of 45 surgically treated cases with emphasis on tumors with osteoblastoma-like features. Arch Pathol Lab Med 2009;133(10):1587–93.
4. Gómez García EB, Knoers NV. Gardner's syndrome (familial adenomatous polyposis): a cilia-related disorder. Lancet Oncol 2009;10(7):727–35.
5. Alexander AA, Patel AA, Odland R. Paranasal sinus osteomas and Gardner's syndrome. Ann Otol Rhinol Laryngol 2007;116(9):658–62.
6. Eller R. Common fibro-osseous lesions of the paranasal sinuses. Otolaryngol Clin North Am 2006;39(3):585–600.
7. Hallberg OE, Begley JW. Origin and treatment of osteomas of the paranasal sinuses. Arch Otolaryngol 1950;51(5):750–60.
8. Cutilli BJ, Quinn PD. Traumatically induced peripheral osteoma. Report of a case. Oral Surg Oral Med Oral Pathol 1992;73(6):667–9.
9. Nielsen GP, Rosenberg AE. Update on bone forming tumors of the head and neck. Head Neck Pathol 2007;1(1):87–93.
10. Fu YS, Perzin KH. Non-epithelial tumors of the nasal cavity, paranasal sinuses, and nasopharynx. A clinicopathologic study. II. Osseous and fibro-osseous lesions, including osteoma, fibrous dysplasia, ossifying fibroma, osteoblastoma, giant cell tumor, and osteosarcoma. Cancer 1974;33(5):1289–305.
11. Koivunen P, Löppönen H, Fors AP, et al. The growth rate of osteomas of the paranasal sinuses. Clin Otolaryngol Allied Sci 1997;22(2):111–4.
12. Larrea-Oyarbide N, Valmaseda-Castellón E, Berini-Aytés L, et al. Osteomas of the craniofacial region. Review of 106 cases. J Oral Pathol Med 2008;37(1):38–42.

13. Zouloumis L, Lazaridis N, Maria P, et al. Osteoma of the ethmoidal sinus: a rare case of recurrence. Br J Oral Maxillofac Surg 2005;43(6):520–2.
14. Bosshardt L, Gordon RC, Westerberg M, et al. Recurrent peripheral osteoma of mandible: report of case. J Oral Surg 1971;29(6):446–50.
15. Gibson T, Walker FM. Large osteoma of the frontal sinus; a method of removal to minimize scarring and prevent deformity. Br J Plast Surg 1951;4(3):210–7.
16. Eckel W, Palm D. Statistical and roentgenological studies on some problems of osteoma of the paranasal sinuses. Arch Ohren Nasen Kehlkopfheilkd 1959;174: 440–57 [in German].
17. Schick B, Steigerwald C, el Rahman el Tahan A, et al. The role of endonasal surgery in the management of frontoethmoidal osteomas. Rhinology 2001; 39(2):66–70.
18. Seiberling K, Floreani S, Robinson S, et al. Endoscopic management of frontal sinus osteomas revisited. Am J Rhinol Allergy 2009;23(3):331–6.
19. Castelnuovo P, Valentini V, Giovannetti F, et al. Osteomas of the maxillofacial district: endoscopic surgery versus open surgery. J Craniofac Surg 2008;19(6): 1446–52.
20. Brodish BN, Morgan CE, Sillers MJ. Endoscopic resection of fibro-osseous lesions of the paranasal sinuses. Am J Rhinol 1999;13(2):111–6.
21. Chiu AG, Schipor I, Cohen NA, et al. Surgical decisions in the management of frontal sinus osteomas. Am J Rhinol 2005;19(2):191–7.
22. Dubin MG, Kuhn FA. Preservation of natural frontal sinus outflow in the management of frontal sinus osteomas. Otolaryngol Head Neck Surg 2006;134(1):18–24.
23. Bignami M, Dallan I, Terranova P, et al. Frontal sinus osteomas: the window of endonasal endoscopic approach. Rhinology 2007;45(4):315–20.
24. Ledderose GJ, Betz CS, Stelter K, et al. Surgical management of osteomas of the frontal recess and sinus: extending the limits of the endoscopic approach. Eur Arch Otorhinolaryngol 2010. Available at: http://www.ncbi.nlm.nih.gov/pubmed/ 20848118. Accessed January 06, 2011.
25. Jurlina M, Janjanin S, Melada A, et al. Large intracranial intradural mucocele as a complication of frontal sinus osteoma. J Craniofac Surg 2010;21(4):1126–9.
26. Akay KM, Ongürü O, Sirin S, et al. Association of paranasal sinus osteoma and intracranial mucocele—two case reports. Neurol Med Chir (Tokyo) 2004;44(4): 201–4.
27. Baykul T, Heybeli N, Oyar O, et al. Multiple huge osteomas of the mandible causing disfigurement related with Gardner's syndrome: case report. Auris Nasus Larynx 2003;30(4):447–51.
28. Rawe SE, VanGilder JC. Surgical removal of orbital osteoma: case report. J Neurosurg 1976;44(2):233–6.
29. Tsai C, Ho C, Lin C. A huge osteoma of paranasal sinuses with intraorbital extension presenting as diplopia. J Chin Med Assoc 2003;66(7):433–5.
30. Gerbrandy SJF, Saeed P, Fokkens WJ. Endoscopic and trans-fornix removal of a giant orbital-ethmoidal osteoma. Orbit 2007;26(4):299–301.
31. Osma U, Yaldiz M, Tekin M, et al. Giant ethmoid osteoma with orbital extension presenting with epiphora. Rhinology 2003;41(2):122–4.
32. Lin C, Lin Y, Kang B. Middle turbinate osteoma presenting with ipsilateral facial pain, epiphora, and nasal obstruction. Otolaryngol Head Neck Surg 2003; 128(2):282–3.
33. Mansour AM, Salti H, Uwaydat S, et al. Ethmoid sinus osteoma presenting as epiphora and orbital cellulitis: case report and literature review. Surv Ophthalmol 1999;43(5):413–26.

34. Naraghi M, Kashfi A. Endonasal endoscopic resection of ethmoido-orbital osteoma compressing the optic nerve. Am J Otolaryngol 2003;24(6):408–12.
35. Nabeshima K, Marutsuka K, Shimao Y, et al. Osteoma of the frontal sinus complicated by intracranial mucocele. Pathol Int 2003;53(4):227–30.
36. Summers LE, Mascott CR, Tompkins JR, et al. Frontal sinus osteoma associated with cerebral abscess formation: a case report. Surg Neurol 2001;55(4):235–9.
37. Shady JA, Bland LI, Kazee AM, et al. Osteoma of the frontoethmoidal sinus with secondary brain abscess and intracranial mucocele: case report. Neurosurgery 1994;34(5):920–3 [discussion: 923].
38. Park MC, Goldman MA, Donahue JE, et al. Endonasal ethmoidectomy and bifrontal craniotomy with craniofacial approach for resection of frontoethmoidal osteoma causing tension pneumocephalus. Skull Base 2008;18(1):67–72.
39. Savić DL, Djerić DR. Indications for the surgical treatment of osteomas of the frontal and ethmoid sinuses. Clin Otolaryngol Allied Sci 1990;15(5):397–404.
40. Smith ME, Calcaterra TC. Frontal sinus osteoma. Ann Otol Rhinol Laryngol 1989; 98(11):896–900.
41. Neel HB, McDonald TJ, Facer GW. Modified Lynch procedure for chronic frontal sinus diseases: rationale, technique, and long-term results. Laryngoscope 1987; 97(11):1274–9.
42. Goodale RL, Montgomery WW. Experiences with the osteoplastic anterior wall approach to the frontal sinus: case histories and recommendations. AMA Arch Otolaryngol 1958;68(3):271–83.
43. Weber R, Draf W, Kratzsch B, et al. Modern concepts of frontal sinus surgery. Laryngoscope 2001;111(1):137–46.
44. Busch RF. Frontal sinus osteoma: complete removal via endoscopic sinus surgery and frontal sinus trephination. Am J Rhinol 1992;6(4):139–43.
45. Menezes CO, Davidson TM. Endoscopic resection of a sphenoethmoid osteoma: a case report. Ear Nose Throat J 1994;73(8):598.
46. Draf W, Weber R. Endonasal micro-endoscopic pansinus operation in chronic sinusitis. I. Indications and operation technique. Am J Otolaryngol 1993;14(6): 394–8.
47. Gross WE, Gross CW, Becker D, et al. Modified transnasal endoscopic Lothrop procedure as an alternative to frontal sinus obliteration. Otolaryngol Head Neck Surg 1995;113(4):427–34.
48. Metson R, Gliklich RE. Clinical outcome of endoscopic surgery for frontal sinusitis. Arch Otolaryngol Head Neck Surg 1998;124(10):1090–6.
49. Kikawada T, Fujigaki M, Kikura M, et al. Extended endoscopic frontal sinus surgery to interrupted nasofrontal communication caused by scarring of the anterior ethmoid: long-term results. Arch Otolaryngol Head Neck Surg 1999;125(1): 92–6.
50. Draf W. Endonasal micro-endoscopic frontal sinus surgery: the fulda concept. Operative Techniques in Otolaryngology Head and Neck Surgery 1991;2(4): 234–40.
51. Timperley D, Banks C, Robinson D, et al. Lateral frontal sinus surgical access after endoscopic lothrop. International Forum of Allergy and Rhinology, in press.

Fibrous Dysplasia of the Sphenoid and Skull Base

Moran Amit, MD[a], Dan M. Fliss, MD[a], Ziv Gil, MD, PhD[b],*

KEYWORDS

- Fibrous dysplasia • Skull base • Sphenoid • Natural history
- Decompression

Key Points: FIBROUS DYSPLASIA OF THE SPHENOID AND SKULL BASE

- Symptomatic patients with optic nerve (ON) involvement can safely be managed by an endonasal surgery directed toward partial decompression of the optic canal.

- Asymptomatic patients with radiologic evidence of ON encasement can be safely managed conservatively with repeated ophthalmologic examinations and long-term radiologic follow-up.

- Although deterioration of vision with time is rare, signs of cranial nerve dysfunction should prompt surgical intervention.

EBM Question	Level of Evidence	Grade of Recommendation
What is natural history of vision in untreated disease?	3a	C
What is the visual outcome of optic nerve decompression?	3a	C

Fibrous dysplasia (FD) is a benign, slowly growing fibro-osseous disease. The histologic process is the replacement of normal bone with various degrees of fibrous tissue and immature woven bone. The disease can involve a single bone (monostotic variant) or multiple bones (polyostotic variant). McCune-Albright syndrome (MAS) is a separate

---

Disclosures: This study was supported in part by funding grants from the US-Israel Binational Science Foundation (2007312) and the Morasha/Heritage Program of the Israel Science Foundation (1680/08) to Ziv Gil.
[a] Department of Otolaryngology Head and Neck Surgery, Tel Aviv Sourasky Medical Center, Tel Aviv University, Tel Aviv, Israel
[b] Head and Neck Surgery Unit, Department of Otolaryngology Head and Neck Surgery, Tel Aviv Sourasky Medical Center, Tel Aviv University, 6 Weitzman Street, Tel Aviv 64239, Israel
* Corresponding author.
E-mail address: ziv@baseofskull.org

Otolaryngol Clin N Am 44 (2011) 891–902
doi:10.1016/j.otc.2011.06.004
0030-6665/11/$ – see front matter © 2011 Elsevier Inc. All rights reserved.

disease entity that is related to FD. It includes polyostotic involvement, hyperfunctional endocrinopathies (precocious puberty, hyperthyroidism, or acromegaly), and skin discoloration (café au-lait).[1,2] Various phenotypes of MAS have been described.

EPIDEMIOLOGY OF FIBROUS DYSPLASIA

FD accounts for 5% to 10% of all bone tumors. Monostotic FD (MFD) is 6- to 10-fold more prevalent than polyostotic FD (PFD), and MAS is less common than the two. There is no gender predilection, and most cases of MFD present in the first 3 decades of life, whereas PFD and MAS tend to present earlier in childhood. Bone involvement varies and is usually unilateral, including mostly ribs and femur, whereas craniofacial involvement occurs in 50% to 100% of patients with the polyostotic form and in 10% with the monostotic variant.[3,4] Among patients with skull lesions, the frontal bones are most commonly involved, followed by the sphenoid, ethmoid, parietal, temporal, and occipital bones.[5] Advanced imaging methodologies demonstrated that ethmoid involvement is the most common, followed by the sphenoid and frontal bones.[6,7] As such, the skull base is the most common site of involvement when the pathology involves the craniofacial skeleton.

PATHOPHYSIOLOGY OF FIBROUS DYSPLASIA

Macroscopically, intramedullary tumors are well circumscribed and vary greatly in size. Large lesions can expand and distort the bone. Microscopically, FD comprises irregular trabeculae of woven immature bone, depicted as Chinese characters, surrounded by normal bone and invested within a cellular fibrous stroma with osteoblast progenitor cells resembling fibroblasts.

Since its first description by Lichtenstein in 1938 as a "perverted activity of the specific bone-forming mesenchyme,"[8] great advancement has been made in our understanding of the pathophysiology of FD. In these tumors, the differentiation of bone marrow stromal cells is arrested, and the immature cells proliferate, giving rise to the fibro-osseous masses that make up FD.[9] The molecular etiology, which leads to the arrest in differentiation, is a somatic missense mutation in the gene GNAS1 on chromosome 20.[10] This gene encodes the alpha subunit of a stimulatory G protein-coupled receptor, Gsα. In FD tumors cells, there is a single amino acid replacement of arginine with either cysteine or histidine, which causes inhibition of the intrinsic GTPase activity of the Gsα protein. This process leads to constitutive, ligand-independent activation and accumulation of cAMP. In bone, it is as if the stromal cells are under constant stimulation, similar to the effect of a parathyroid hormone. A similar mechanism is responsible for the extraskeletal manifestations, including constitutive activation of skin melanocytes, ovarian stimulation, and hyperthyroidism. It was suggested that the burden of mutated cells in FD is influenced by growth factors and hormones and frequently declines with age, resulting in tumor arrest.[11]

CLINICAL FEATURES OF FIBROUS DYSPLASIA

The clinical picture of skull base FD depends on the pathologic bone's compressive effectagainst adjacent structures. Patients are usually asymptomatic and present with a painless bony enlargement leading to deformity and asymmetry.[12,13] The most common symptoms are facial asymmetry, bone mass, blurred vision, headache, epiphora, eyelid position abnormalities, loss of visual field, diplopia, sinusitis, epistaxis, and hearing loss (**Box 1**).[14] It is most convenient to categorize patients into 3 distinctive groups according to their symptoms: asymptomatic, headaches,

---

Box 1
Signs and symptoms of fibrous dysplasia

Facial asymmetry (86%)

Mass (64%)

Epiphora (7%)

Headache (20%)

Blurred vision (24%)

Eyelid position abnormalities (10%)

Loss of visual field (8%)

Diplopia (8%)

Sinusitis (8%)

Epistaxis (3%)

Hearing loss (3%)

---

and cranial nerve compression. Asymptomatic patients are usually diagnosed during the evaluation of head trauma or radicular cervical spine symptoms.[15]

EVALUATION AND RADIOLOGIC WORKUP FOR FIBROUS DYSPLASIA

Diagnosis of MFD is generally based on clinical symptoms and radiological evaluation. In contrast, patients with PFD often require bone biopsy for histopathologic diagnosis. Radiological workup usually includes computed tomography (CT) and magnetic resonance imaging (MRI). Scintigraphy can be used to assess the disease burden throughout the body. CT is efficient for assessing cranial nerve entrapment and ON compression (**Fig. 1**).[16,17] Three-dimensional bone reconstruction with helical CT gives optimal visualization of the extent of dysplastic bone in the skull base.[18] FD has characteristic appearances on CT: a ground-glass pattern (50%), a homogeneously dense pattern (25%), and cystic variety (20%).[19] On MRI, the signal intensity on T1- and T2-weighted images depends on several factors, including the amount of bone trabeculation and the degree of cellularity.[20,21] Characteristically, lesions show low-signal intensity and well-demarcated borders on both T1- and T2-weighted images (**Fig. 2**). The hypointense signal intensity on T2-weighted images is caused by the numerous bony trabeculae.[18] Single photon emission CT has been reported to be sensitive in detecting the boundaries of FD involvement.[22]

NATURAL HISTORY OF FIBROUS DYSPLASIA

The natural history of FD has an important impact on decision making. It had been thought that FD becomes inactive after puberty,[23–26] but recent publications reported that FD can occur after adolescence and progress into adulthood.[20] Similarly, it was shown that one-third of the surgically treated patients had recurrence during adulthood.[7,27,28] Although most tumors in patients with MFD arrest after puberty, there is a higher rate of disease progression in PFD, and most patients with MAS will demonstrate progression of bone lesion during adulthood.[29] Lee and colleagues[30] described 38 patients with sphenoid region FD who did not undergo surgery; 80% of the optic canals in the patients aged younger than 30 years were encased by FD, whereas only 44% of the optic canals in the patients aged 30 years

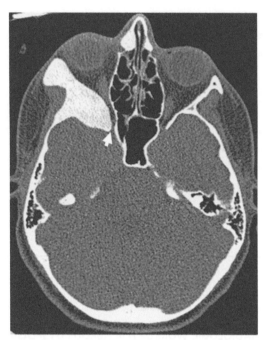

Fig. 1. ON compression by fibrous dysplasia of the sphenoid bone. Axial CT image showing narrowing of the optic canal caused by enlarged lesser wing of sphenoid (*arrow*).

or older were encased, suggesting a regression in the disease. The incidence of malignant transformation of FD is 0.4%.[26,31] Sarcomatous transformation, mainly to fibrosarcoma or osteosarcoma, was reported in patients undergoing radiation therapy.[32]

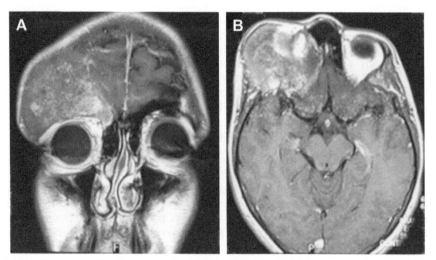

Fig. 2. (*A*) Coronal and (*B*) axial postcontrast T1-weighted MR images showing right supraorbital low intensity mass with characteristic ground glass appearance. Inhomogeneous areas might represent fibrous tissue, cyst formation, or hemorrhage.

MEDICAL TREATMENT OF FIBROUS DYSPLASIA

In the absence of level-1 evidence, most data on the management of FD rely on expert opinion. Some studies investigated the utility of pharmaceutical treatment for FD.[33] One of the most extensively investigated therapies is bisphosphonates, which inhibit osteoclastic bone resorption.[34,35] Intravenous administration of pamidronate for 2 years was reported to induce rapid improvement in the degree of pain and disfigurement among 13 children with FD,[36] but this treatment was stopped because of a severe increase in bone mass index in those patients. In another study, half of the patients with MFD reported significant improvement in symptoms and mass growth after 22 months.[37] High-dose oral bisphosphonate was also reported to improve symptoms.[38] Response is usually monitored with bone turnover markers, such as serum alkaline phosphatase and urinary hydroxyproline, which are not useful for diagnosis. Serial radiographs have also been used to assess treatment response, but the results are inconsistent. One study demonstrated response to treatment by the filling of osteolytic lesions and cortical thickening, whereas others showed no radiological response.[33,39] Local bone mineral density has been found to be more consistent than serial radiographs in the monitoring of the response to treatment.[37] The major drawback of these works is the short period of follow-up and the selection bias of easier cases (ie, those without major disfiguring lesions and neuropathies). The latter usually skip the consultation with endocrinologists and present directly to neurosurgeons, plastic surgeons, otolaryngologists, or ophthalmologists, depending on clinical picture. Hence, double blind, placebo-controlled, randomized trials are needed to demonstrate the efficacy of bisphosphonates for the palliation and control of tumor bulk. The role of steroid treatment has been described in a few cases and its effect was limited in time.[40–42] It is recommended for use only in cases of acute visual deterioration with the intent of buying time before surgery.

SURGICAL INTERVENTION FOR FIBROUS DYSPLASIA

It is generally acceptable that asymptomatic sphenoid FD does not necessitate biopsy or surgery, and that a clinico-radiological follow-up is sufficient. Surgery is advocated once patients become symptomatic (eg, cranial neuropathies, pain, or disfigurement). On the other hand, management of asymptomatic patients with radiologic evidence of ON compression is debatable (see later discussion).

Surgeons must be familiar with the course of disease and rate of recurrence before a decision is made regarding surgery. Earlier series mainly used debulking and recontouring of facial bones in patients with cosmetic deformity caused by FD. As a result, the reported recurrence rate was up to 25%.[24,43,44] Because of such a high rate of recurrence after curettage, some investigators recommended radical excision and reconstruction for patients with orbital hypertelorism, dystopia, exophthalmos, or grotesque orbitofacial deformity.[45] Because extensive removal of FD is associated with a low rate of tumor recurrence, this type of surgery was especially recommended for children with low predicted surgical morbidity and for symptomatic patients.[46]

Recent advances in surgical technique have enabled more radical surgery and immediate reconstruction with good aesthetic and functional outcomes. As a result, the more conservative surgeries became less popular for the management of FD.[14,47] Based on their experience with 28 patients with craniofacial FD (CFD) Chen and Noordhoff suggested classification of the disease status into 4 surgical groups: zone 1, which includes the fronto-orbital, zygomatic, and upper maxillary regions; zone 2, which represents the hair-bearing cranium; zone 3, which includes the central cranial base; and zone 4, which involves the teeth-bearing regions of the maxillary alveolus and mandible.[48] They suggested a total tumor excision in zone 1 and conservative excision for lesions involving zones 2, 3, and 4. They recommended treatment only in the presence of symptoms for patients with lesions in zone 3.[15,48] The surgical approach is determined according to the location and extent of the disease. Most lesions can be approached anteriorly, either endoscopically or via transfacial approaches or coronal flap.[49–51] Solitary lesions of the ethmoidal, frontal, and sphenoid area can be safely resected by endonasal surgery.[7]

OPTIC NERVE INVOLVEMENT IN FIBROUS DYSPLASIA

A major issue in the management of patients with CFD is the role of optic canal decompression. In FD of the sphenoid bone, the rate of ON involvement is 50% to 90%.[52] The degree of ON involvement varies between mild impingement of the nerve to a totally encased nerve.[30] Cutler and colleagues[53] reported 87 patients with CFD, all of whom had ON involvement; 83% of the nerves had more than 50% ON encasement. The high rate of ON involvement and the potential risk of visual impairment as a result of nerve compression have led many surgeons to suggest prophylactic decompression of the ON in patients who are asymptomatic. The proponents of prophylactic surgery claim that unfavorable postoperative results were obtained in patients who had long-standing ON compression and that they had atrophic optic discs.[54–56] Another of their arguments was the rapid course of permanent visual deterioration in patients with radiologic evidence of ON encasement,[41,42,52,56–58] with visual impairment having been reported in 20% to 80% of patients with ON encasement.[43,59–61] Based on these results, Chen and colleagues[52] argued that if the optic canal is radiologically involved, one-third of the patients will have visual deficits and up to two-thirds will report some degree of visual disturbance.

In contrast to earlier reports, later cross-sectional studies challenged the high risk of ON atrophy in patients with CFD. In 2 sentinel articles, Lee and colleagues[30] and Culter and colleagues[53] reported that the vast majority of asymptomatic patients with CFD will maintain normal vision despite radiological evidence of ON involvement. These unexpected results described normal vision even in patients with total encasement of the optic canal. The majority of the patients in this group had MAS; and Cutler and colleagues[53] found significant correlation between increased growth hormone secretion and optic neuropathy (a relative risk of 3.8). ON compression can also result from secondary lesions, including cystic fibrous dysplasia, mucoceles, hemorrhage, and aneurismal bone cysts.[62]

ON decompression is not risk free, and cases of blindness and visual deterioration in asymptomatic patients have been reported.[61,63–65] The high risk of ON injury was attributed to the sensitivity of the compressed nerve to surgical insult.[66] Therefore, partial decompression of the optic canal was suggested for reducing the pressure on the nerve in symptomatic patients. The vision of such patients is expected to remain stable or improve after surgery. Even in patients with bilateral FD and unilateral optic neuropathy, the risk for blindness in decompression of the asymptomatic side must be given serious consideration.

The authors analyzed all the relevant cases published in the English literature to evaluate the efficacy and outcome of decompression in asymptomatic patients with optic canal narrowing caused by FD. A PubMed, Google scholar, and the Cochrane Central Register of Controlled Trials search was conducted through September 2010 using the Medical Subject Headings terms (fibrous dysplasia) AND (orbit OR vision OR visual OR optic OR exophthalmus OR diplopia OR proptosis). Reference lists of selected articles were manually searched for additional publications. Two reviewers (M.A. and Z.G.) independently reviewed titles and abstracts of search results to determine if the content was related to the study outcome. Studies that were identified for potential inclusion were assessed by using a priori inclusion criteria and standardized forms.

The inclusion criteria according to the study design were any randomized controlled trial, a prospective cohort, a retrospective cohort, case-control study designs, case reports, and case series. Criteria for study population inclusion were

1. Preoperative or postoperative histopathology diagnosis of FD
2. Radiologically demonstrated optic canal narrowing
3. Pretreatment and posttreatment visual status (based on visual fields and visual acuity or patient visual status report)
4. At least 4 months of follow-up.

All studies were rated by the Oxford evidence-based guidelines. The authors excluded publications that did not report numeric data in a format conducive to a meta-analysis. The investigators of the included articles were contacted by email for further information about patient follow-up and outcome. Publications in a language other than English could not be translated because of resource constraints and were excluded. The two reviewers independently abstracted information from each included study. Discrepancies were resolved by discussion and consensus.

The search of the literature resulted in 248 articles. One hundred sixty-seven available full texts were screened. Forty-six relevant articles were reviewed. Seventeen articles were excluded because of insufficient data or for not meeting the inclusion criteria, 1 article was excluded because of duplicate publication,[52] and 1 article in the conservative treatment group was excluded because of high-dose bisphosphonate treatment.[38] A total of 198 patients were included, 88 of whom (44%) had MAS.[7,43,46,52,60,62,63,67–86] The average age was 20 years (range 8–40), and the average follow-up was 67 months (range 6–228). Gender details were not available for the FD subgroups. A total of 295 ONs were involved, representing 92 cases of bilateral involvement and 5 cases of recurrence. One-half of the patient population (n = 99) had ON decompression (71 therapeutic and 28 prophylactic), and the other half were followed conservatively with serial radiographs and ophthalmologic evaluations.

Symptomatic patients who underwent surgical decompression had a 65% rate of stable vision during long-term follow-up. In asymptomatic patients, the results of this meta-analysis revealed stable vision in 87% of patients undergoing optic canal decompression and in 97% of the patients that did not undergo surgery ($P<.001$). There was no significance difference in the age and mean follow-up period between the two groups of patients.

DISCUSSION

Craniofacial FD is a genetic nonhereditary disease that has a benign course in most patients. It can progress beyond puberty, and there is no correlation between age and clinical course. Cranial nerve involvement is rare in this population. The presence of a mucocele or bone cyst may increase the risk of visual deterioration caused by ON compression.

The absence of level-1 evidence on the management of patients with FD makes it difficult to decide on the optimal patient management. Because disease progression is not inevitable, it is difficult to predict which patient will progress to have a debilitating disease. Considering the risk of surgical injury to the ON together with the unknown course of the disease, the possibility of an adverse outcome must be considered seriously before operating on asymptomatic patients. The accumulated experience reported in the literature revealed in the authors' meta-analysis shows no difference in the visual deterioration rate between prophylactically and therapeutically decompressed nerves. The significantly lower rate of adverse visual outcome in conservatively treated patients suggests that performing decompression in asymptomatic patients unnecessarily puts the ON at risk. Moreover, the prevalence of visual deterioration during follow-up is rare, even in patients with MAS who usually exhibit a more aggressive course of disease.

In conclusion, published data and the authors' meta-analysis suggest that symptomatic patients with ON involvement can safely be managed by an endonasal surgery directed toward partial decompression of the optic canal. On the other hand, asymptomatic patients with radiologic evidence of ON encasement should be managed conservatively with repeated ophthalmologic examinations and long-term radiologic follow-up. Although deterioration of vision with time is rare in this population, signs of cranial nerve dysfunction should prompt surgical intervention.

Grade B recommendation, Level 3 evidence

EBM Question	Author's reply
What is natural history of vision in untreated disease?	Asymptomatic optic nerve encasement is often stable for many years (97% mean follow-up 67 months) with visual loss often associated with other factors such as increased growth hormone secretion (a relative risk of 3.8) and other secondary lesions such cystic fibrous dysplasia, mucoceles, hemorrhage, and aneurismal bone cysts
What is the visual outcome of optic nerve decompression?	65% stable vision in symptomatic patients undergoing surgery and 87% of prophylactically treated patients at mean follow-up at 67 months

ACKNOWLEDGMENTS

Esther Eshkol is thanked for editorial assistance.

REFERENCES

1. Albright F, Butler M, Hamptom A, et al. Syndrome characterized by osteitis fibrosa disseminata, areas of pigmentation and endocrine dysfunction with precocious puberty in females. N Engl J Med 1937;216:727.
2. McCune D, Bruch H. Osteodystrophia fibrosa: report of a case in which the condition was combined with precocious puberty, multiple pigmentation of the skin and hyperthyroidism. Am J Dis Child 1937;52:745.
3. Eversole LR, Sabes WR, Rovin S. Fibrous dysplasia: a nosologic problem in the diagnosis of fibro-osseous lesions of the jaws. J Oral Pathol 1972;1:189.
4. Windholz F. Cranial manifestations of fibrous dysplasia of bone; their relation to leontiasis ossea and to simple bone cysts of the vault. Am J Roentgenol Radium Ther 1947;58:51.
5. Vinken PJ, Bruyn GW. Neuroretinal degenerations. Amsterdam. New York: North-Holland Pub. Co.; American Elsevier Pub. Co; 1972.
6. Abdelkarim A, Green R, Startzell J, et al. Craniofacial polyostotic fibrous dysplasia: a case report and review of the literature. Oral Surg Oral Med Oral Pathol Oral Radiol Endod 2008;106:e49.

7. Lustig LR, Holliday MJ, McCarthy EF, et al. Fibrous dysplasia involving the skull base and temporal bone. Arch Otolaryngol Head Neck Surg 2001;127:1239.
8. Lichtenstein L. Polyostotic fibrous dysplasia. Arch Surg 1938;36:874.
9. Bianco P, Riminucci M, Majolagbe A, et al. Mutations of the GNAS1 gene, stromal cell dysfunction, and osteomalacic changes in non-McCune-Albright fibrous dysplasia of bone. J Bone Miner Res 2000;15:120.
10. Robey PG, Bianco P. The role of osteogenic cells in the pathophysiology of Paget's disease. J Bone Miner Res 1999;14(Suppl 2):9.
11. Cohen MM Jr, Howell RE. Etiology of fibrous dysplasia and McCune-Albright syndrome. Int J Oral Maxillofac Surg 1999;28:366.
12. Becelli R, Perugini M, Cerulli G, et al. Surgical treatment of fibrous dysplasia of the cranio-maxillo-facial area. Review of the literature and personal experience form 1984 to 1999. Minerva Stomatol 2002;51:293.
13. Yavuzer R, Bone H, Jackson IT. Fronto-orbital fibrous dysplasia. Orbit 2000;19:119.
14. Rahman AM, Madge SN, Billing K, et al. Craniofacial fibrous dysplasia: clinical characteristics and long-term outcomes. Eye (Lond) 2009;23:2175.
15. Adada B, Al-Mefty O. Fibrous dysplasia of the clivus. Neurosurgery 2003;52:318.
16. Chen YR, Wong FH, Hsueh C, et al. Computed tomography characteristics of nonsyndromic craniofacial fibrous dysplasia. Chang Gung Med J 2002;25:1.
17. Tehranzadeh J, Fung Y, Donohue M, et al. Computed tomography of Paget disease of the skull versus fibrous dysplasia. Skeletal Radiol 1998;27:664.
18. MacDonald-Jankowski DS. Fibro-osseous lesions of the face and jaws. Clin Radiol 2004;59:11.
19. Brown EW, Megerian CA, McKenna MJ, et al. Fibrous dysplasia of the temporal bone: imaging findings. AJR Am J Roentgenol 1995;164:679.
20. Jee WH, Choi KH, Choe BY, et al. Fibrous dysplasia: MR imaging characteristics with radiopathologic correlation. AJR Am J Roentgenol 1996;167:1523.
21. Yano M, Tajima S, Tanaka Y, et al. Magnetic resonance imaging findings of craniofacial fibrous dysplasia. Ann Plast Surg 1993;30:371.
22. Nakahara T, Fujii H, Hashimoto J, et al. Use of bone SPECT in the evaluation of fibrous dysplasia of the skull. Clin Nucl Med 2004;29:554.
23. Leeds N, Seaman WB. Fibrous dysplasia of the skull and its differential diagnosis. A clinical and roentgenographic study of 46 cases. Radiology 1962;78:570.
24. Ramsey HE, Strong EW, Frazell EL. Fibrous dysplasia of the craniofacial bones. Am J Surg 1968;116:542.
25. Ricalde P, Horswell BB. Craniofacial fibrous dysplasia of the fronto-orbital region: a case series and literature review. J Oral Maxillofac Surg 2001;59:157.
26. Tanaka Y, Tajima S, Maejima S, et al. Craniofacial fibrous dysplasia showing marked involution postoperatively. Ann Plast Surg 1993;30:71.
27. Davies ML, Macpherson P. Fibrous dysplasia of the skull: disease activity in relation to age. Br J Radiol 1991;64:576.
28. Katz BJ, Nerad JA. Ophthalmic manifestations of fibrous dysplasia: a disease of children and adults. Ophthalmology 1998;105:2207.
29. Kusano T, Hirabayashi S, Eguchi T, et al. Treatment strategies for fibrous dysplasia. J Craniofac Surg 2009;20:768.
30. Lee JS, FitzGibbon E, Butman JA, et al. Normal vision despite narrowing of the optic canal in fibrous dysplasia. N Engl J Med 2002;347:1670.
31. Schwartz DT, Alpert M. The malignant transformation of fibrous dysplasia. Am J Med Sci 1964;247:1.
32. Goaz PW, White SC. Oral radiology: principles and interpretation. 3rd edition. St Louis (MO): Mosby; 1994.

33. Chapurlat RD. Medical therapy in adults with fibrous dysplasia of bone. J Bone Miner Res 2006;21(Suppl 2):P114.

34. Devogelaer JP. Treatment of bone diseases with bisphosphonates, excluding osteoporosis. Curr Opin Rheumatol 2000;12:331.

35. Glorieux FH, Rauch F. Medical therapy of children with fibrous dysplasia. J Bone Miner Res 2006;21(Suppl 2):P110.

36. Makitie AA, Tornwall J, Makitie O. Bisphosphonate treatment in craniofacial fibrous dysplasia–a case report and review of the literature. Clin Rheumatol 2008;27:809.

37. Kos M, Luczak K, Godzinski J, et al. Treatment of monostotic fibrous dysplasia with pamidronate. J Craniomaxillofac Surg 2004;32:10.

38. Chao K, Katznelson L. Use of high-dose oral bisphosphonate therapy for symptomatic fibrous dysplasia of the skull. J Neurosurg 2008;109:889.

39. Plotkin H, Rauch F, Zeitlin L, et al. Effect of pamidronate treatment in children with polyostotic fibrous dysplasia of bone. J Clin Endocrinol Metab 2003;88:4569.

40. Bland LI, Marchese MJ, McDonald JV. Acute monocular blindness secondary to fibrous dysplasia of the skull: a case report. Ann Ophthalmol 1992;24:263.

41. Osguthorpe JD, Gudeman SK. Orbital complications of fibrous dysplasia. Otolaryngol Head Neck Surg 1987;97:403.

42. Weisman JS, Hepler RS, Vinters HV. Reversible visual loss caused by fibrous dysplasia. Am J Ophthalmol 1990;110:244.

43. Edgerton MT, Persing JA, Jane JA. The surgical treatment of fibrous dysplasia. With emphasis on recent contributions from cranio-maxillo-facial surgery. Ann Surg 1985;202:459.

44. Jaffe HL. Tumors and tumorous conditions of the bones and joints. Philadelphia: Lea & Febiger; 1958.

45. Ozek C, Gundogan H, Bilkay U, et al. Craniomaxillofacial fibrous dysplasia. J Craniofac Surg 2002;13:382.

46. Maher CO, Friedman JA, Meyer FB, et al. Surgical treatment of fibrous dysplasia of the skull in children. Pediatr Neurosurg 2002;37:87.

47. Valentini V, Cassoni A, Marianetti TM, et al. Craniomaxillofacial fibrous dysplasia: conservative treatment or radical surgery? A retrospective study on 68 patients. Plast Reconstr Surg 2009;123:653.

48. Chen YR, Noordhoff MS. Treatment of craniomaxillofacial fibrous dysplasia: how early and how extensive? Plast Reconstr Surg 1991;87:799.

49. Ferguson BJ. Fibrous dysplasia of the paranasal sinuses. Am J Otolaryngol 1994;15:227.

50. Ikeda K, Suzuki H, Oshima T, et al. Endonasal endoscopic management in fibrous dysplasia of the paranasal sinuses. Am J Otolaryngol 1997;18:415.

51. Ragab MA, Mathog RH. Surgery of massive fibrous dysplasia and osteoma of the midface. Head Neck Surg 1987;9:202.

52. Chen YR, Breidahl A, Chang CN. Optic nerve decompression in fibrous dysplasia: indications, efficacy, and safety. Plast Reconstr Surg 1997;99:22.

53. Cutler CM, Lee JS, Butman JA, et al. Long-term outcome of optic nerve encasement and optic nerve decompression in patients with fibrous dysplasia: risk factors for blindness and safety of observation. Neurosurgery 2006;59:1011.

54. Calderon M, Brady HR. Fibrous dysplasia of bone with bilateral optic foramina involvement. Am J Ophthalmol 1969;68:513.

55. Donoso LA, Magargal LE, Eiferman RA. Fibrous dysplasia of the orbit with optic nerve decompression. Ann Ophthalmol 1982;14:80.

56. Kurokawa Y, Sohma T, Tsuchita H, et al. Hemorrhage into fibrous dysplasia following minor head injury–effective decompression for the ophthalmic artery and optic nerve. Surg Neurol 1989;32:421.
57. Papay FA, Morales L Jr, Flaharty P, et al. Optic nerve decompression in cranial base fibrous dysplasia. J Craniofac Surg 1995;6:5.
58. Sevel D, James HE, Burns R, et al. McCune-Albright syndrome (fibrous dysplasia) associated with an orbital tumor. Ann Ophthalmol 1984;16:283.
59. Chen YR, Fairholm D. Fronto-orbito-sphenoidal fibrous dysplasia. Ann Plast Surg 1985;15:190.
60. Kurimoto M, Endo S, Onizuka K, et al. Extradural optic nerve decompression for fibrous dysplasia with a favorable visual outcome. Neurol Med Chir (Tokyo) 1996; 36:102.
61. Sassin JF, Rosenberg RN. Neurological complications of fibrous dysplasia of the skull. Arch Neurol 1968;18:363.
62. Michael CB, Lee AG, Patrinely JR, et al. Visual loss associated with fibrous dysplasia of the anterior skull base. Case report and review of the literature. J Neurosurg 2000;92:350.
63. Edelstein C, Goldberg RA, Rubino G. Unilateral blindness after ipsilateral prophylactic transcranial optic canal decompression for fibrous dysplasia. Am J Ophthalmol 1998;126:469.
64. Finney HL, Roberts TS. Fibrous dysplasia of the skull with progressive cranial nerve involvement. Surg Neurol 1976;6:341.
65. Moore AT, Buncic JR, Munro IR. Fibrous dysplasia of the orbit in childhood. Clinical features and management. Ophthalmology 1985;92:12.
66. Lei P, Bai H, Wang Y, et al. Surgical treatment of skull fibrous dysplasia. Surg Neurol 2009;72(Suppl 1):S17.
67. Goisis M, Biglioli F, Guareschi M, et al. Fibrous dysplasia of the orbital region: current clinical perspectives in ophthalmology and cranio-maxillofacial surgery. Ophthal Plast Reconstr Surg 2006;22:383–7.
68. Abe T, Satoh K, Wada A. Optic nerve decompression for orbitofrontal fibrous dysplasia: recent development of surgical technique and equipment. Skull Base 2006;16:145–55.
69. Panda NK, Parida PK, Sharma R, et al. A clinicoradiologic analysis of symptomatic craniofacial fibro-osseous lesions. Otolaryngol Head Neck Surg 2007;136:928–33.
70. Cruz AA, Constanzi M, de Castro FA, et al. Apical involvement with fibrous dysplasia: implications for vision. Ophthal Plast Reconstr Surg 2007;23:450–4.
71. Tan YC, Yu CC, Chang CN, et al. Optic nerve compression in craniofacial fibrous dysplasia: the role and indications for decompression. Plast Reconstr Surg 2007; 120:1957–62.
72. Tabrizi R, Ozkan BT. Craniofacial fibrous dysplasia of orbit. J Craniofac Surg 2008;19:1532–7.
73. Liakos GM, Walker CB, Carruth JA. Ocular complications in craniofacial fibrous dysplasia. Br J Ophthalmol 1979;63:611–6.
74. Misra M, Mohanty AB, Rath S. Orbital reconstruction in fibrous dysplasia–a case report. Indian J Ophthalmol 1990;38:39–41.
75. McCluskey P, Wingate R, Benger R, et al. Monostotic fibrous dysplasia of the orbit: an unusual lacrimal fossa mass. Br J Ophthalmol 1993;77:54–6.
76. Dowler JG, Sanders MD, Brown PM. Bilateral sudden visual loss due to sphenoid mucocele in Albright's syndrome. Br J Ophthalmol 1995;79:503–4.
77. Bocca G, de Vries J, Cruysberg JR, et al. Optic neuropathy in McCune-Albright syndrome: an indication for aggressive treatment. Acta Paediatr 1998;87:599–600.

78. Horgan MA, Delashaw JB, Dailey RA. Bilateral proptosis: an unusual presentation of fibrous dysplasia. Br J Neurosurg 1999;13:335–7.
79. Thomas C, Mahapatra AK, Joy MJ, et al. Craniofacial surgery in Oman: a preliminary study of 10 cases. J Craniofac Surg 2001;12:247–52.
80. Jan M, Dweik A, Destrieux C, et al. Fronto-orbital sphenoidal fibrous dysplasia. Neurosurgery 1994;34:544–7 [discussion: 547].
81. Sharma RR, Mahapatra AK, Pawar SJ, et al. Symptomatic cranial fibrous dysplasias: clinico-radiological analysis in a series of eight operative cases with follow-up results. J Clin Neurosci 2002;9:381–90.
82. Fujimoto A, Tsuboi K, Ishikawa E, et al. Surgery improves vision and cosmetic appearance of an adult patient with fibrous dysplasia of the frontal bone. J Clin Neurosci 2004;11:95–7.
83. Movassaghi K, Janecka I. Optic nerve decompression via mid-facial translocation approach. Ann Plast Surg 2005;54:331–5.
84. Tajima T, Tsubaki J, Ishizu K, et al. Case study of a 15-year-old boy with McCune-Albright syndrome combined with pituitary gigantism: effect of octreotide-long acting release (LAR) and cabergoline therapy. Endocr J 2008;55:595–9.
85. Yang X, Guo Z, Mu X, et al. A lateral approach at the upper corner of the orbit in fronto-orbital fibrous dysplasia: less invasive and more effective approach for morphologic reconstruction and optic functional restoration. J Craniofac Surg 2009;20(Suppl 2):1831–5.
86. Bibby K, McFadzean R. Fibrous dysplasia of the orbit. Br J Ophthalmol 1994;78: 266–70.

Orbit and Orbital Apex

Dan Robinson, BIT, BCom, FRACS[a], Geoff Wilcsek, MB BS, FRANZCO[b],
Raymond Sacks, MBBCH, FCS (SA) ORL, FRACS, MMed (ORL)[c,*]

KEYWORDS

- Orbital apex • Traumatic optic neuropathy
- Graves orbitopathy • Orbital pseudotumor
- Orbital decompression • Optic nerve decompression
- Ophthalmology

EBM Question	Level of Evidence	Grade of Recommendation
Does vision improve following decompression of traumatic and tumor pathology?	2b	B
What is optimal timing of endoscopic decompression?	4	C

Pathology affecting the orbit and orbital apex is diverse and heterogeneous. Many of the differential pathologies require management in a multidisciplinary team involving both otolaryngology and ophthalmology. This article discusses the differential pathologies. Emphasis has been placed on Graves orbitopathy (GO), traumatic optic neuropathy (TON), and the indications for decompression in each. The differential diagnosis for a lesion within the orbit and orbital apex is diverse (**Box 1**). The presentation, investigation, and appropriate management of these conditions is discussed with emphasis on TON and GO.

The authors have nothing to disclose.
[a] Department of Otolaryngology Head and Neck Surgery, Royal Prince Alfred Hospital, University of Sydney, 50 Missenden Road, Camperdown, Sydney, New South Wales 2050, Australia
[b] Oculoplastics Unit, Department of Ophthalmology, The Prince of Wales Hospital, University of New South Wales, Barker Street, Randwick, Sydney, New South Wales 2031, Australia
[c] Department of Otolaryngology Head and Neck Surgery, Concord Hospital, Hornsby Hospital, University of Sydney, Hospital Road, Concord, Sydney, New South Wales 2139, Australia
* Corresponding author. ENT Centre, Suite 12, The Madison, 25-29 Hunter Street, Hornsby Hospital, Palmerston Road, Hornsby, New South Wales 2077, Australia.
E-mail address: rsacks@optusnet.com.au

Otolaryngol Clin N Am 44 (2011) 903–922
doi:10.1016/j.otc.2011.06.011
0030-6665/11/$ – see front matter © 2011 Elsevier Inc. All rights reserved.

oto.theclinics.com

Box 1
Differential diagnosis of lesions in orbit and orbital apex

- Infectious
  - Bacterial
  - Fungal
- Inflammatory
  - GO
  - Idiopathic orbital inflammation
  - Granulomatous
- Traumatic
- Neoplastic benign
  - Vascular
  - Neural
  - Fibro-osseous
- Neoplastic malignant
  - Lymphoma
  - Epithelial
  - Nonepithelial
  - Secondary

INFECTIOUS SINUSITIS
Bacterial

Bacterial infections of the orbit are classified by the Chandler classification. Any infection that is Chandler classification 4 or more, which is within the orbit, requires prompt surgical drainage. The treatment for Chandler classification 3, which is a subperiosteal abscess, is more controversial with some investigators advocating a trial of medical therapy before offering surgery.

Investigations

All patients with a suspected subperiosteal abscess should have a CT scan with contrast of their paranasal sinuses to confirm the diagnosis and to visualize the anatomy of the sinuses.[1] If it is suspected the patient has intracranial complications, they should proceed to having an MRI scan.

Organisms most commonly found in subperiosteal abscess are *Streptococci*, *Staphylococci*, and *Bacteroides*.[1]

Treatment

All patients with an orbital complication of sinusitis require antibiotics. The authors propose the use of a third-generation cephalosporin and an antistaphylococcal agent. The controversial decision is whether the patient needs to have surgical drainage of their abscess and the proposed timing of surgery.

The authors use Garcia and Harris criteria for a trial of nonsurgical management. The criteria that must be satisfied are:[2]

- Age of patient less than 9 years old
- No visual compromise

- Medial abscess of modest or small size
- No intracranial or frontal sinus involvement.

If these criteria are not met, the patient requires drainage with endoscopic as the preferred method. The use of age as a requirement for consideration for drainage is because patients over age 9 years have an increased incidence of infections that are refractory to antibiotics.[2]

The authors advocate that if an endonasal approach to medial subperiosteal abscess is not possible, drainage should be performed using a transcaruncular approach rather than a Lynch incision. This approach is typically performed by an ophthalmologist with oculoplastic training. It has the advantage over the Lynch incision of gaining more linearly direct access to the medial subperiosteal space, avoiding a skin incision and resulting scar, as well as avoiding injury to the adjacent trochlear and superior oblique attachment.

If the patient worsens clinically, they are given prompt surgical drainage.

Fungal Sinusitis

Fungal sinusitis can be subdivided into invasive and noninvasive fungal sinusitis. Invasive fungal sinusitis requires prompt aggressive surgical debridement. Noninvasive fungal sinusitis that has developed an orbital complication can be initially treated medically before surgical drainage. The details of the diagnosis and treatment modalities of fungal sinusitis are beyond the scope of this paper.

INFLAMMATORY DISEASES OF THE ORBIT
GO

GO is the most common extrathyroidal manifestation of Graves disease.[3] Although GO occurs in Graves disease, it may also manifest in patients who have no history of Graves disease, patients who are euthyroid, or in patients who have autoimmune thyroiditis.[4] Approximately 20% of patients who have GO are euthyroid.

Pathogenesis

The exact pathogenesis of GO is incompletely understood.[4] GO is an autoimmune disease that macroscopically has evidence of an increase in the volume of extraocular muscles, increased orbital fat volume due to adipogenesis, and inflammation of orbital connective tissue with a varying degree of cicatrisation of the orbital contents.[3,5] Histopathological changes include an infiltration of T lymphocytes and macrophages in the orbital tissue as well as increased production of hydrophilic glycosaminoglycans.[6,7] The most likely explanation for these findings in GO is an antigen shared between the thyroid and the orbital tissue. This antigen is most likely the thyrotropin receptor antigen; however, there are several other antigens that may potentially be associated with GO.[5,8] Regardless of what the antigenic stimuli is, T cells recognize the antigen and initiate an inflammatory response.[3]

Multiple mechanisms may increase in intraconal volume in GO. The first and most common finding in patients with GO is increased extraocular muscle mass and an increase in orbital fat mass (**Fig. 1**). The second possible finding is an increase in muscle mass without an increase in the fat mass. The third possibility and rarest finding is of a normal muscle mass and increased fat mass.[9]

The orbit is bounded posteriorly by its bony canal and anteriorly by the tarsoligamentous diaphragm. Therefore, any increase in intraconal volume results in a rise in intraorbital pressure. The rise in pressure at the apex leads to decreased venous

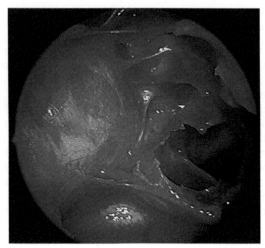

Fig. 1. Intraoperative GO. Note the bulging periorbital fat and increased muscle mass of the medial rectus.

drainage resulting in chemosis and periorbital edema, causing further enlargement of the orbital volume.[10]

Epidemiology

Approximately 50% of patients who have Graves disease will develop orbital manifestations.[5] There is a genetic predisposition to the development of GO; family members of patients with GO have a higher chance of manifesting the disease.[5]

Graves disease is more common in females and, therefore, GO is more common in females. However, when GO is present in a male it is usually more severe and progressive than in a female.[11] GO is rare in the pediatric population.[12]

There is a strong relationship between the development of GO and smoking. Smokers develop GO more frequently and the disease is more severe in smokers with the active phase of the disease having a longer time course. Development of GO in smokers is dose dependant.[13] Smokers have a sevenfold increased risk of developing extraocular muscle fibrosis in GO.[5]

Natural history

GO has two distinct phases: active and inactive. Active disease lasts for 6 months to 3 years.[14] During the active phase inflammation, fibrosis and adipogenesis occur resulting in changing signs on physical examination. Inactive disease is defined as the period of the disease where the signs do not progress during a 6 month period. The signs and symptoms of GO can also regress without treatment in up to two-thirds of cases.[15]

In general, medical treatment is offered during the active phase, surgical treatment is offered during the inactive phase.[4]

Clinical features of GO

The most common clinical signs that are apparent are[16]

- Eyelid retraction, present in 90% of cases
- Proptosis, present in 60% of cases
- Extraocular muscle dysfunction, present in 40% of cases.

Other features that commonly occur are

- Eyelid and periorbital edema
- Conjunctival injection and chemosis
- Corneal erosions and superior limbic keratitis.

Optic neuropathy is a less common but very important feature of GO, occurring in 2% to 8% of cases.[17] Optic neuropathy should be suspected when there is decreased best-corrected visual acuity and diagnosed when associated with constricted visual field, red desaturation, and a relative afferent pupillary defect.

The authors consider GO to be severe when vision is at risk. Visual loss in GO occurs in these scenarios:

1. Optic neuropathy. Most commonly secondary to pressure on the nerve due to increased intraorbital volume. It is important to note that fibrosis of the annulus of Zinn and enlargement of the extraocular muscles at the orbital apex can result in optic neuropathy without significant proptosis.[9] More uncommonly, optic neuropathy can be the result of stretch on the optic nerve rather than pressure. On imaging, the posterior sclera is seen to tent at an angle of 90 degrees.
2. Corneal exposure and scarring. Proptosis combined with lid retraction causes poor lid closure or lagophthalmos. This can lead to corneal ulceration, corneal scarring, or perforation of the globe.

Investigations
All patients who are being considered for active surgical intervention should have a CT scan of their paranasal sinuses. Signs that may be apparent on CT scan include excess retroorbital fat, enlargement of the extraocular muscles, and crowding of the orbital apex.[17] As an adjunct to a CT scan, MRI allows for more accurate visualization of the optic nerve and extraocular muscles, as well as potential determination of disease activity.[11] Although imaging is not required in all cases of GO, it should be strongly considered when intervention is being planned.

Treatment
Given the high natural resolution rate of GO and the high degree of cases that remain static, the clinician needs to be mindful that a significant proportion of patients will not require treatment.[15]

Medical treatment
Steroids are a proven treatment for GO and are especially efficacious during the active phase of the disease. Steroids are effective for reducing the extraocular muscle dysfunction and for reducing the optic neuropathy. However, they are not as effective when it comes to reduction in proptosis.[4] Recurrence of the disease both when the steroid is tapered and during steroid therapy is a problem in GO. The major drawback of steroid therapy is that it is often required for several months with associated long-term effects of steroid use.

External beam radiotherapy delivered to the orbital tissue is also a proven treatment modality in patients with active GO. The rationale for the use of radiotherapy in GO is the antiinflammatory effect that it has, as well as the radiosensitivity of the lymphocytes in the orbital tissue.[4] With the exception of extraocular muscle involvement and proptosis, most of the manifestations of GO respond well to radiotherapy. Patients who have severe hypertension or diabetic retinopathy should not be offered radiotherapy due to their risk of developing microvascular abnormalities associated with the treatment.

Multiple immunotherapy drugs, such as tumor necrosis factor inhibitor, are under investigation for their treatment effect in GO. Once their treatment effect has been established, they may become part of the medical treatment for GO.[18]

Surgery

In GO, there is often a mismatch between the volume of the orbit contents and the volume of the bony cavity. This can be addressed surgically by a fat decompression or a bony decompression of one or multiple orbital walls.[17] Bony decompression is applicable across a wider range of GO patients, so orbital fat decompression will not be discussed further.

The indications recommend for bony orbital decompression in GO are[4,11]

- Optic neuropathy
- Contraindication to or inability to tolerate medical treatment of optic neuropathy
- Clinically severe proptosis that causes exposure keratopathy or is cosmetically unacceptable.

The authors recommend endoscopic medial wall decompression, without exposing the optic nerve in the sphenoid sinus and with teasing out of orbital fat, combined with a balanced decompression of the lateral wall with excision of a portion of the infero-lateral fat pad. Once the bone is removed, the periorbita is opened to allow the fat to prolapse.

The most common risk of this operation is diplopia. The diplopia may be transient or require strabismus surgery. According to the literature, the risk of diplopia varies—ranging from 10% to as high as 60%.[4,19] Multiple techniques have been examined to reduce the postoperative diplopia; however, there is no one technique that has demonstrated consistently superior results.[19] Significant decompression of the orbital floor is associated with the highest rate of postoperative diplopia.

When there is evidence of optic neuropathy, the authors recommend medial wall decompression with exposure of the optic nerve in the sphenoid sinus and without optic nerve sheath fenestration. There is a higher degree of postoperative diplopia in patients who have intervention for optic neuropathy associated with GO than in patients who do not have intervention.[19]

In some cases of GO, there is progression of symptoms after surgery. In these instances, prior surgery is not a contraindication to further decompression and can be associated with an improvement in outcome.[14]

Measures of treatment success

The measurement of proptosis as a marker of success with an exophthalmometer is widely used preoperatively and postoperatively. The degree of reduction that can be obtained via an endoscopic technique alone is 3.5 mm, on average.[10] When external approaches are used or combined with endoscopic approaches, the average reduction in proptosis is 7.4 mm.[20] However, when correlating the degree of proptosis reduction with the visual acuity outcomes or diplopia outcomes, there appears to be little correlation.[10]

After surgical decompression, visual acuity improves. However, given the heterogeneity of the surgical indications, it is difficult to give an accurate number for the expected degree of improvement.[10] In cases of GO-associated optic neuropathy, the improvement that is seen in visual acuity postoperatively is as high as 89%.[21] Analyzing success in patients who have the procedure performed for cosmetic or reconstructive reasons is difficult given the lack of comparability between studies.

The authors consider the chance of success in an appropriately selected patient to be very high from a cosmetic or reconstructive point of view.

Idiopathic Orbital Inflammation

Idiopathic orbital inflammation comprises about 10% of orbital lesions.[22] The exact cause of this condition is unknown. It is a diagnosis of exclusion, with lymphoma being the most important differential to exclude.

Idiopathic orbital inflammation is otherwise known as orbital pseudotumor. It is further divided into acute and sclerosing subtypes.

Clinical

Patients present with a variety of symptoms and signs, including:

- Proptosis
- Diplopia
- Pain
- Lid swelling
- Ptosis
- Chemosis.

Investigations

Imaging of the orbit is required in the form of CT scan and/or MRI. The appearance of orbital pseudotumor is a nonspecific orbital mass.[22]

The authors advocate a low threshold to biopsy idiopathic orbital inflammation, especially if there is a doubt as to the diagnosis or the clinical course is not typical for the disease. Twenty-five percent of patients that are appropriately treated with steroids will recur and these patients require biopsy. When there is isolated lacrimal gland involvement, the authors advocate for a low threshold for biopsy to exclude malignancy, which can have a similar presentation in the lacrimal gland.[23]

Treatment

Idiopathic orbital inflammation is a medical condition that is most commonly treated with and is acutely sensitive to oral steroids. Radiotherapy, chemotherapy, or immunosuppression may be appropriate for the treatment of either refractory acute or sclerosing idiopathic orbital inflammation.[22]

This should be done by a multidisciplinary team involving an ophthalmologist and immunologist. Surgery for treatment of idiopathic orbital inflammation should only be considered in the establishment of the diagnosis or when there is an apical mass causing optic neuropathy. In this instance, an apical decompression is used as temporizing measure while awaiting the effect of medical treatment.

Granulomatous

Granulomatous diseases can present in the orbit. These include Wegener granulomatosis, sarcoidosis, and, less commonly, Churg-Strauss disease and xanthogranuloma.

The presentation of granulomatous diseases of the orbit is of a nonspecific orbital inflammation and involvement. The diagnosis is made by a combination of inflammatory markers, imaging, and a biopsy if there is doubt as to the diagnosis.

Once diagnosis for these lesions has been made, it is managed by a multidisciplinary team using immunosuppression. Again, in the scenario of progressive optic neuropathy, an apical decompression is occasionally needed to temporize while awaiting the effect of medical treatment.

TRAUMATIC

Up to 5% of cases of head injury affect some portion of the visual system with 0.5% to 1.5% of patients having TON.[24,25] The morbidity of TON can be devastating for the patient.[26] The exact mechanism of TON associated with head injury is unknown and both direct and indirect mechanisms have been proposed as potential causes.[27]

Presently there are no accepted guidelines for the treatment of TON. Various modalities have been examined, including conservative management, steroids, and surgery. No intervention has proved more beneficial than observation. However, despite the lack of evidence for different treatment modalities, there is justification in offering these patients treatment provided that the risks of the treatment do not exacerbate morbidity and that the patient is adequately informed of these risks.[28]

Mode of Injury

There are two accepted modes of injury in TON: direct and indirect. Direct TON is the result of anatomic disruption of the optic nerve. The potential causes for this include penetrating eye injury, iatrogenic transaction, fracture of an adjacent bone, or hematoma.

Indirect TON is the result of the transmission of force to the optic canal and orbital apex from a distant site usually as a result of blunt trauma.[29] The initial force is believed to cause a shockwave that is transmitted directly to the optic canal, causing damage to the optic nerve. In many cases of TON, the injury is a mixture of both direct and indirect injury.[29]

Anatomic studies have determined that the force that is initiated at the forehead is focused at the optic canal because the dural sheath of the optic nerve is densely adherent to the periosteum of the optic canal. Force transmitted to the skull is transmitted directly to the optic canal and via the dura to the optic nerve. As a result, the segment of the optic nerve within the optic canal is the most susceptible to injury.[30,31]

Pathophysiology

The exact pathophysiology of TON is unknown and it is probably multifactorial. Two types of injury have been proposed to occur in TON: primary and secondary. Primary injury causes irreversible damage to a proportion of the retinal ganglion cells. Retinal ganglion cells are cells within the optic nerve that are involved in transmitting information from the eye to the visual centers in the brain. In response to this initial traumatic insult, the optic nerve begins to swell. The vasculature of the optic nerve is pial and the swelling causes a compartment syndrome resulting in ischemia to the nerve.[32] This compartment syndrome is then followed by a reduction in blood supply to the optic nerve. The resultant hypoxia causes an upregulation of oxygen free radicals and rise in intracellular calcium with resultant apoptosis.[29,32] This apoptosis is referred to as the secondary injury. A proportion of this secondary injury is reversible, which accounts for the improvement in vision in TON. The basis for treatment in TON is preservation of the cells that have survived the initial trauma, thus preventing them from undergoing apoptosis as a result of the secondary injury.

Epidemiology

The average age of patients who have TON is late 20s to early 30s, and the majority of patients are male. The mode of delivery is usually force applied directly to the forehead.[26] The most common cause of optic neuropathy in adults is motor vehicle accidents followed by falls. The degree of force required to cause TON varies greatly and it can manifest as a result of minor trauma.[27,33] In the pediatric population the majority of cases are caused by falls.[34]

Clinical

TON is a clinical diagnosis using the history of the trauma and examination. The history of the trauma can range from motor vehicle accidents to minor trauma, such as a fall.[27] A subset of patients who present with TON are obtunded because of their head injury. Due to the difficulty in assessing these patients, their diagnosis is usually delayed.[35] The features of TON are:[29]

1. Ocular involvement, unilateral or bilateral
2. Relative afferent papillary defect on ipsilateral side, except in cases of bilateral traumatic optic neuropathy
3. Reduction in visual acuity
4. Decreased color vision
5. Variable visual field defects
6. Optic disc that appears normal in most cases, except where injury is anterior to the entry point of the retinal vessels with associated optic disc swelling
7. Optic atrophy in the period following injury, usually becoming apparent after 3 weeks.

Not all of the previous findings may be present in a patient with TON, which may make the diagnosis difficult. However, all cases of TON have a reduction in vision and a relative afferent papillary defect provided the patient has a unilateral lesion.[26]

Investigations

Imaging is the mainstay of investigation for a patient with TON. Most institutions perform a CT scan as a routine investigation before considering intervention. The CT scan will aid in the diagnosis of an underlying fracture of the bones adjacent to the optic nerve. However, the utility of the imaging modality is under debate because there is no correlation between the findings on CT scan and the visual loss or prognosis associated with the patient's vision.[36]

Additional imaging includes an MRI; however, this is not routinely performed in all institutions. The utility of MRI has not been extensively examined and, in many patients with TON who have other significant injuries, obtaining an MRI may be impractical.[37]

Visual evoked potential (VEP) has been described as an adjunctive investigation in patients who are obtunded from their initial injury. The VEP has been demonstrated to be predictive of long-term outcome.[37] When the VEP is absent, recovery of vision is unlikely. When the VEP amplitude is within 50% of the normal side, the patient might have a favorable outcome. It is reasonable to conclude that VEP can be used to aid in the diagnosis of TON in the obtunded patient. At present, however, it is cumbersome to move the required equipment to the bedside.

Treatment of Traumatic Optic Neuropathy

Treatment options for TON are:

1. Conservative
2. Steroids
3. Surgery
4. Surgery and steroids.

Treatment data for TON is difficult to collect given the nature of the condition and understandable controversy surrounding randomizing a patient with no vision to conservative management.

The classification of successful treatment of TON varies in the literature with the larger series accepting between greater than or equal to two lines of improvement in visual acuity and greater than or equal to three lines of improvement in acuity.[26,33]

Conservative management

Conservative management of TON has a variable rate of improvement. The reported rate of improvement in the conservative arm of studies ranges from 40% to 60%.[29] Although these figures would seem to advocate conservative management in all cases, it is important to remember that the majority of patients who undergo conservative management are more likely to have a good baseline visual acuity, which then correlates to better long-term results.

Medical intervention

Medical treatment for TON traditionally involves the use of a high dose of corticosteroids with the aim that they will suppress the inflammatory response that causes the optic nerve injury.[38] The rationale for steroids in TON is drawn from multiple sources, including animal data gathered while looking at spinal cord trauma outcomes and studies of acute spinal cord trauma patients who achieved a better outcome when steroids were given in the first 8 hours.[39–41] Mechanisms through which high-dose steroids may influence the outcome in TON are:

1. Improved blood flow locally
2. Antioxidant activity causing a reduction in oxygen free radicals production and decreasing subsequent lipid peroxidation.[29,42]

The dose that has been investigated varies between studies—ranging from 60 mg to 7 g of corticosteroid per day.

The International Optic Nerve Trauma Study (IONTS) was a multicenter trial that looked at 133 patients with TON and treated them on a nonrandom basis to receive either no treatment, steroids, or optic nerve decompression. The study found that the improvement in vision in the steroid arm of treatment was 52%. However, when compared with the other interventions of steroids and surgery, this result was not found to be significant.[26] The Cochrane Review on the use of steroids in TON found that documented improvement rates with steroids varied from 44% to 62%.[29]

Subgroup analysis in the IONTS looking at the different dose regimens demonstrated no significant difference in patients who received higher dose steroids versus patients who received the lower dose steroids.[26] The study concluded that there is no evidence to support use of high-dose steroids over low-dose steroids in TON. However, the power of IONTS may not be adequate to support such a conclusion.

The duration of steroid application between studies is highly variable. Some studies began to taper the dose of steroids after 11 days[43] and others ceased steroids completely after 9 days of treatment.[33]

In conclusion, the Cochrane review on the use of steroids in TON found no strong evidence to support the use of steroids.[29] When applying this treatment effect clinically, the IONTS concluded that the use of steroids for the treatment of TON should be individualized to the clinical scenario.[26]

Surgical intervention

Surgical treatment of TON involves endoscopic decompression of the optic nerve.[44] The results from surgery are variable across different studies ranging from 9.5% through to 55%.[26,33,45]

In the IONTS, 32% of patients improved with surgery. In this study, there was significant variation in the surgical procedure performed. They ranged from endoscopic to open procedures, and the timing of the surgery differed from less than 24 to 72 hours after injury. When analyzing the results of surgery, the investigators found no significant difference between surgery versus steroids versus conservative treatment. One of the major confounders in this study is the surgery arm had many patients who were initially treated with steroids and failed to respond. As a result, a significant amount of patients in the surgery arm had more significant injury than patients in the steroid arm, which could ultimately lower the expected response in the surgery arm.[26]

One of the larger series examined the results of 237 patients with TON. They were offered surgery in a nonrandom fashion and those treated with surgery demonstrated an improvement in vision of 55%. However, this was not significant when compared with the treatment effect of steroids, which was 51%.[33]

Combined modality

Although no trial has been done comparing surgery alone and steroids in combination with surgery, the majority of patients who get surgery have received combined modality therapy.[26,33] One of the larger series attempted to determine if there was significant benefit from offering combined modality treatment but was unable to demonstrate an improved result.[33]

Prognostic Factors

Baseline visual acuity is the most important predictor of outcome in TON.[29] Patients with no light perception at presentation have the worst outcome regardless of intervention.[26] One of the larger studies demonstrated that patients who present with gradual visual loss have a better outcome than patients who present with complete blindness.[33]

The prognosis for direct and indirect injury to the optic nerve differs. Direct injury to the optic nerve where there has been significant penetration or transection carries a poor prognosis regardless of whether or not there is active intervention. The patients with direct optic nerve injury are more likely to present with sudden visual loss. Conversely, indirect injury to the optic nerve has demonstrated that prognosis may potentially be improved with intervention.[46]

Multiple studies have demonstrated a statistically significant improvement in prognosis if the surgery is performed less than 7 days, versus greater than 7 days, after the initial insult.[33,34,43] However, there are also studies that found no significant difference in outcome related to timing of surgery.[36]

The presence of a fracture in a bone adjacent to the optic nerve has been examined in several studies. The findings of many studies are contradictory. Some have shown that a fracture was a significant predictor in outcome and others have found it not significant (**Figs. 2** and **3**).[26,47]

The IONTS demonstrated that there was no significant difference in outcome when comparing patient age or gender.[26,36]

Safety of Intervention

The safety of very high doses of steroids is controversial. In the absence of statistically significant treatment data, a clinician must ask whether the safety profile of the treatment being offered is worth the risk to the patient.[48] This topic has been examined in the National Acute Spinal Cord Injury Study (NASCIS) trials. In NASCIS-II, patients who received megadoses of steroids for 24 hours were noted to have a nonstatistically significant increase in the rate of gastrointestinal bleeding.[40] In NASCIS-III, patients who received megadoses of steroids for greater than 48 hours had a nonstatistically significant increase in their rate of sepsis and pneumonia.[41] The conclusion of these trials on the safety of very high doses of steroids is that they are relatively safe; however, may be associated with complications.

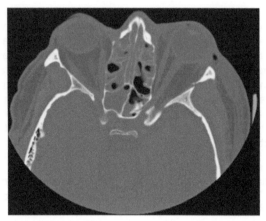

Fig. 2. CT scan of a fracture through the left orbital apex impinging the optic nerve.

The Corticosteroid Randomization After Significant Head Injury (CRASH) trial examined efficacy and safety of high dose steroids for 48 hours in the setting of head trauma. This trial was terminated early because of a higher risk of death in the steroid arm of the trial. The cause of death in the steroid treatment arm has not been determined.[49] Considering that between 40% and 72% of cases of TON are associated with head injury, the results of this trial must be taken into consideration.[50] Therefore, in the setting of head injury, there needs to be adequate consent regarding the potential complications of high-dose steroids.

The safety of optic nerve decompression has been examined in many studies. One of the larger cohorts of 176 patients has demonstrated that no patient experienced worsening vision associated with their procedure. Complications that were reported in this series include one injury to the ophthalmic artery, three cases of cerebrospinal fluid leak, and two cases of an intraorbital infection.[33] Other complications that have been reported include a case of intraoperative carotid artery bleeding.[43] Overall, endoscopic decompression is regarded as a relatively safe procedure to undertake provided the operating surgeon has the required experience.[51]

Several studies have indicated a need for a randomized, controlled trial to investigate the treatment of TON. However, given the low incidence of the condition and the obvious dilemmas surrounding randomizing treatment, it is less likely that such a trial will take place.[26]

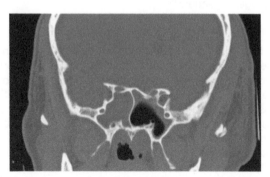

Fig. 3. CT scan of a fracture through the left orbital apex impinging the optic nerve.

Recommendations for Treatment of TON

IONTS concluded that the treatment of TON should be made on an individual patient basis.[26] The data concerning different modes of intervention is inconclusive and it is entirely appropriate that each case be managed on its merits.

The indications that the authors recommend for the use of high-dose steroids are:

1. Clinical evidence of TON
2. No contraindication to steroids
3. Injury less than 72 hours ago.

If the patient has had a closed head injury, steroids should be given in consultation with a neurosurgeon and intensive care specialist, and informed consent discussed with the relatives of the patient to ensure they understand the risks and benefits for steroids in this setting. Steroids may be of benefit after 72 hours; however, the benefit is significantly reduced if initiation is delayed.

The indications for optic nerve decompression remain controversial.[48] The indications to operate that the authors recommend are similar to those offered by Rajiniganth[43]:

1. Failure for vision to improve after 72 hours of high-dose steroid therapy
2. Progressive visual loss during steroid therapy
3. Complete blindness with CT scan evidence of optic nerve compression
4. Contraindication to steroids with progressive visual loss
5. Loss of vision with CT scan evidence of fracture or hematoma impinging on optic nerve.

The authors recommend that the patient have an optic nerve decompression with incision of the optic nerve sheath. The nerve sheath is incised for its entire length within the sphenoid. This operation should be performed by a surgeon who is familiar with the anatomy and capable of treating any potential complications of the intervention (**Figs. 4** and **5**).

NEOPLASTIC BENIGN
Vascular Malformations

Vascular lesions of the orbit are probably a continuous spectrum rather than distinct entities.[52] They range from the lymphangioma being no flow, orbital varices that are

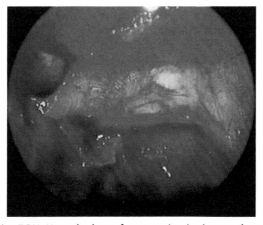

Fig. 4. Intraoperative TON. Note the bony fragment impinging on the optic nerve.

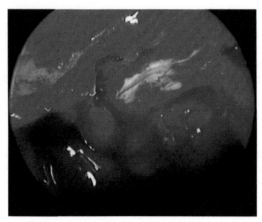

Fig. 5. Intraoperative TON. Optic nerve sheath fenestration.

low flow, to arteriovenous malformations. Excisional surgery for any of these lesions is often unsatisfactory at best; however, orbital apical decompressive surgery can play an invaluable role. For example, lymphangiomas can have a course of recurrent hemorrhage. If the lesion has no capsule and infiltrates through many orbital structures, decompression at the time of optic neuropathy is a more useful surgical tool than attempted excisional surgery. Vascular malformations of the orbit should be managed by a multidisciplinary team, including an ophthalmologist.

Neural

Neural-derived tumors of the orbit and orbital apex consist of glioma, neurofibroma, schwannoma, and meningioma. Presentation is dependent on tumor type and position within the orbit, with neurofibroma and schwannoma tending to be more anterior and meningioma and glioma typically being retrobulbar. In general, management of these lesions should be by a multidisciplinary team.

Meningiomas affecting the orbital apex are either derived from the optic nerve sheath or sphenoid wing lesions. Optic nerve sheath meningiomas share the blood supply of the optic nerve via pial vessels. Therefore, biopsy or removal of the meningioma causes damage to the blood supply of the optic nerve, resulting in visual loss. Subsequently, management of optic nerve meningioma should be conservative unless the patient has complete visual loss. In patients who have a meningioma and have complete visual loss, any resection must be done with consideration for the potential risk of visual loss in the contralateral eye. Several nerve fibers from the opposite optic nerve extend several millimeters anterior to the chiasm along the contralateral optic nerve, known as von Willebrand knee.[53] Any resection of the optic nerve should spare a few millimeters anterior to the chiasm so as not to affect the contralateral superolateral visual field that is represented in von Willebrand knee.

Fibro-Osseous

Fibro-osseous lesions that affect the optic nerve and orbit have the same pathology as fibro-osseous lesions that affect the paranasal sinuses. These lesions are primarily fibrous dysplasia, ossifying fibroma, and osteoma.

Fibrous Dysplasia

Fibrous dysplasia presents as either monostotic or polyostotic fibrous dysplasia. McCune-Albright syndrome is a subset of polyostotic fibrous dysplasia. Treatment for fibrous dysplasia within the orbit should be of an expectant nature, with lesions that are causing compression or symptoms requiring surgery. Asymptomatic stable lesions can be safely observed.

Ossifying Fibroma

Ossifying fibroma is an aggressive lesion that can be locally destructive. When ossifying fibroma is found within the orbit or adjacent, the orbit removal is recommended early as the lesion will likely expand and cause symptoms if it is not already doing so.

Osteoma

Osteomas are benign osseous lesions that grow slowly. They have an increased incidence at the frontoethmoidal suture line and, therefore, may encroach on the orbit (**Figs. 6** and **7**).[54] They may come to the attention of the clinician due to compression of adjacent structures or alternatively as an incidental finding. Given their slow growth, they are more likely to present with a chronic history.[55]

Treatment of Fibro-Osseous Lesions

The symptoms that are caused by fibro-osseous lesions are by mass effect. Specific to the orbit, patients will present with diplopia, epiphora, and, more rarely, a reduction in visual acuity.[55] The other mode of presentation is as an incidental finding.

Removal of the fibro-osseous lesion is recommended under the following circumstances:

- Significant signs or symptoms
- Suspicion of ossifying fibroma
- Suspicion of malignant transformation.

Given their expansive nature, the younger the patient the more likely an ossifying fibroma or osteoma is going to cause problems throughout the patient's life. Therefore, the clinician should have a lower threshold for treating these conditions in the younger population. The prognosis for an improvement in visual acuity following removal of the fibro-osseous lesion is good.[55]

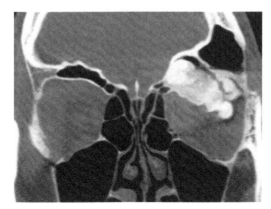

Fig. 6. Osteoma lesion.

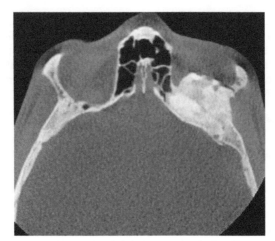

Fig. 7. Osteoma lesion.

NEOPLASTIC MALIGNANT
Lymphoma

Lymphoma typically presents with a painless mass effect in the orbit. MRI shows a highly cellular mass that tends to grow around orbital structures. Biopsy with immunohistochemistry and flow cytometry is required for diagnosis and planning treatment. Treatment depends on stage and tumor type and consists of radiotherapy and/or chemotherapy.

Epithelial

Primary epithelial tumors of the orbit are rare. These tumors most commonly involve the lacrimal gland but can involve any other part of the orbit. Epithelial tumors of the lacrimal gland range from benign pleomorphic adenoma to the highly malignant adenoid cystic carcinoma and squamous cell carcinoma.

Nonepithelial

Rhabdomyosarcoma is the most common primary orbital malignancy of childhood. Rhabdomyosarcoma should be considered in all children who present with progressive proptosis. Other sarcomas, such as liposarcoma and leiomyosarcoma, are rare but can also present in the orbit.

Metastatic

Metastatic tumors can present in the orbit. These include:

- Neuroblastoma
- Leukemia
- Breast carcinoma
- Lung carcinoma
- Prostate carcinoma.

SUMMARY

Pathology occurring in the orbit and orbital apex is diverse and it is important that the clinician has a differential diagnosis to consider, as well as an understanding of the treatment of the more common conditions. Many of these conditions require combined management with an ophthalmologist and are best managed by a multidisciplinary team. Consideration must be given to orbital decompression and optic nerve decompression when appropriate.

Vision does improve following decompression for traumatic and tumor pathology. Level of evidence of recommendation—D.

Timing of surgery should be within 7 days of the injury. Level of recommendation—C.

The current evidence for optic nerve decompression varies from low-powered studies to case control series. There are no randomized control trials covering optic nerve decompression and, given the nature of the condition, it is unlikely a trial with significant power will be produced. For patients with TON and no contraindication to steroids, the authors advocate the use of high-dose steroids. Following failure of steroid treatment or progression of the condition, the authors advocate optic nerve decompression. If a patient has a fracture impinging on the optic nerve, the authors advocate removal of the fragment. Level of recommendation—D.

Timing of the surgery should be within 7 days. Visual outcomes associated with TON decrease if the decompression is performed after 7 days. The authors advocate that the surgery be performed as soon as is practically and medically possible. Level of recommendation—C.

EBM Question	Author's reply
Does vision improve following decompression of traumatic and tumor pathology?	Vision improves after both medical or surgical intervention (Level 2b) and maybe better than no treatment in trauma (Level 3a)
What is optimal timing of endoscopic decompression?	Optimal timing of endoscopic decompression: 1. Failure for vision to improve after 72 hours of high-dose steroid therapy 2. Progressive visual loss during steroid therapy 3. Complete blindness with CT scan evidence of optic nerve compression 4. Contraindication to steroids with progressive visual loss 5. Loss of vision with CT scan evidence of fracture or hematoma impinging on optic nerve. 6. Documented early visual loss in non-traumatic pathology where the natural history of the disease would suggest progression

REFERENCES

1. Fakhri S, Pereira K. Endoscopic management of orbital abscesses. Otolaryngol Clin North Am 2006;39:1037.
2. Garcia GH, Harris GJ. Criteria for nonsurgical management of subperiosteal abscess of the orbit: analysis of outcomes 1988–1998. Ophthalmology 2000; 107:1454.
3. Burch HB, Wartofsky L. Graves' ophthalmopathy: current concepts regarding pathogenesis and management. Endocr Rev 1993;14:747.
4. Bartalena L, Pinchera A, Marcocci C. Management of Graves' ophthalmopathy: reality and perspectives. Endocr Rev 2000;21:168.
5. Eckstein AK, Johnson KT, Thanos M, et al. Current insights into the pathogenesis of Graves' orbitopathy. Horm Metab Res 2009;41:456.
6. Gorman CA. Pathogenesis of Graves' ophthalmopathy. Thyroid 1994;4:379.

7. Weetman AP, Cohen S, Gatter KC, et al. Immunohistochemical analysis of the retrobulbar tissues in Graves' ophthalmopathy. Clin Exp Immunol 1989;75:222.
8. Smith TJ. Pathogenesis of Graves' orbitopathy: a 2010 update. J Endocrinol Invest 2010;33:414.
9. Kazim M, Trokel SL, Acaroglu G, et al. Reversal of dysthyroid optic neuropathy following orbital fat decompression. Br J Ophthalmol 2000;84:600.
10. Leong SC, White PS. Outcomes following surgical decompression for dysthyroid orbitopathy (Graves' disease). Curr Opin Otolaryngol Head Neck Surg 2010; 18:37.
11. Lee HB, Rodgers IR, Woog JJ. Evaluation and management of Graves' orbitopathy. Otolaryngol Clin North Am 2006;39:923.
12. Bartalena L, Baldeschi L, Dickinson AJ, et al. Consensus statement of the European group on Graves' orbitopathy (EUGOGO) on management of Graves' orbitopathy. Thyroid 2008;18:333.
13. Pfeilschifter J, Ziegler R. Smoking and endocrine ophthalmopathy: impact of smoking severity and current vs lifetime cigarette consumption. Clin Endocrinol (Oxf) 1996;45:477.
14. Leung MK, Platt MP, Metson R. Revision endoscopic orbital decompression in the management of Graves' orbitopathy. Otolaryngol Head Neck Surg 2009;141:46.
15. Perros P, Crombie AL, Kendall-Taylor P. Natural history of thyroid associated ophthalmopathy. Clin Endocrinol (Oxf) 1995;42:45.
16. Bartley GB, Fatourechi V, Kadrmas EF, et al. Clinical features of Graves' ophthalmopathy in an incidence cohort. Am J Ophthalmol 1996;121:284.
17. Chu EA, Miller NR, Lane AP. Selective endoscopic decompression of the orbital apex for dysthyroid optic neuropathy. Laryngoscope 2009;119:1236.
18. Bartalena L, Lai A, Sassi L, et al. Novel treatment modalities for Graves' orbitopathy. Pediatr Endocrinol Rev 2010;7(Suppl 2):210.
19. Graham SM, Brown CL, Carter KD, et al. Medial and lateral orbital wall surgery for balanced decompression in thyroid eye disease. Laryngoscope 2003;113:1206.
20. Chu EA, Miller NR, Grant MP, et al. Surgical treatment of dysthyroid orbitopathy. Otolaryngol Head Neck Surg 2009;141:39.
21. Schaefer SD, Soliemanzadeh P, Della Rocca DA, et al. Endoscopic and transconjunctival orbital decompression for thyroid-related orbital apex compression. Laryngoscope 2003;113:508.
22. Mendenhall WM, Lessner AM. Orbital pseudotumor. Am J Clin Oncol 2010;33:304.
23. Harris GJ. Idiopathic orbital inflammation: a pathogenetic construct and treatment strategy: the 2005 ASOPRS Foundation Lecture. Ophthal Plast Reconstr Surg 2006;22:79.
24. Sofferman RA. Sphenoethmoid approach to the optic nerve. Laryngoscope 1981; 91:184.
25. Steinsapir KD, Goldberg RA. Traumatic optic neuropathy. Surv Ophthalmol 1994; 38:487.
26. Levin LA, Beck RW, Joseph MP, et al. The treatment of traumatic optic neuropathy: the International Optic Nerve Trauma Study. Ophthalmology 1999;106:1268.
27. Warner JE, Lessell S. Traumatic optic neuropathy. Int Ophthalmol Clin 1995;35:57.
28. Levin LA, Baker RS. Management of traumatic optic neuropathy. J Neuroophthalmol 2003;23:72.
29. Yu-Wai-Man P, Griffiths PG. Steroids for traumatic optic neuropathy. Cochrane Database Syst Rev 2007;1:CD006032.
30. Anderson RL, Panje WR, Gross CE. Optic nerve blindness following blunt forehead trauma. Ophthalmology 1982;89:445.

31. Gross CE, DeKock JR, Panje WR, et al. Evidence for orbital deformation that may contribute to monocular blindness following minor frontal head trauma. J Neurosurg 1981;55:963.

32. Sarkies N. Traumatic optic neuropathy. Eye 2004;18:1122.

33. Li H, Zhou B, Shi J, et al. Treatment of traumatic optic neuropathy: our experience of endoscopic optic nerve decompression. J Laryngol Otol 2008;122:1325.

34. Gupta AK, Gupta A, Malhotra SK. Traumatic optic neuropathy in pediatric population: early intervention or delayed intervention? Int J Pediatr Otorhinolaryngol 2007;71:559.

35. Yu Wai Man P, Griffiths PG. Surgery for traumatic optic neuropathy. Cochrane Database Syst Rev 2005;4:CD005024.

36. Levin LA, Joseph MP, Rizzo JF 3rd, et al. Optic canal decompression in indirect optic nerve trauma. Ophthalmology 1994;101:566.

37. Warner N, Eggenberger E. Traumatic optic neuropathy: a review of the current literature. Curr Opin Ophthalmol 2010;21:459.

38. Spoor TC, Hartel WC, Lensink DB, et al. Treatment of traumatic optic neuropathy with corticosteroids. Am J Ophthalmol 1990;110:665.

39. Anderson DK, Means ED, Waters TR, et al. Microvascular perfusion and metabolism in injured spinal cord after methylprednisolone treatment. J Neurosurg 1982;56:106.

40. Bracken MB, Shepard MJ, Collins WF, et al. A randomized, controlled trial of methylprednisolone or naloxone in the treatment of acute spinal-cord injury. Results of the Second National Acute Spinal Cord Injury Study. N Engl J Med 1990;322:1405.

41. Bracken MB, Shepard MJ, Holford TR, et al. Administration of methylprednisolone for 24 or 48 hours or tirilazad mesylate for 48 hours in the treatment of acute spinal cord injury. Results of the Third National Acute Spinal Cord Injury Randomized Controlled Trial. National Acute Spinal Cord Injury Study. JAMA 1997;277:1597.

42. Hall ED, Braughler JM. Glucocorticoid mechanisms in acute spinal cord injury: a review and therapeutic rationale. Surg Neurol 1982;18:320.

43. Rajiniganth MG, Gupta AK, Gupta A, et al. Traumatic optic neuropathy: visual outcome following combined therapy protocol. Arch Otolaryngol Head Neck Surg 2003;129:1203.

44. Kountakis SE, Maillard AA, Urso R, et al. Endoscopic approach to traumatic visual loss. Otolaryngol Head Neck Surg 1997;116:652.

45. Li HB, Shi JB, Cheng L, et al. Salvage optic nerve decompression for traumatic blindness under nasal endoscopy: risk and benefit analysis. Clin Otolaryngol 2007;32:447.

46. Carta A, Ferrigno L, Salvo M, et al. Visual prognosis after indirect traumatic optic neuropathy. J Neurol Neurosurg Psychiatry 2003;74:246.

47. Cook MW, Levin LA, Joseph MP, et al. Traumatic optic neuropathy. A meta-analysis. Arch Otolaryngol Head Neck Surg 1996;122:389.

48. Perry JD. Treatment of traumatic optic neuropathy remains controversial [author reply: 1000]. Arch Otolaryngol Head Neck Surg 2004;130:1000.

49. Roberts I, Yates D, Sandercock P, et al. Effect of intravenous corticosteroids on death within 14 days in 10008 adults with clinically significant head injury (MRC CRASH trial): randomised placebo-controlled trial. Lancet 2004;364:1321.

50. Steinsapir KD. Treatment of traumatic optic neuropathy with high-dose corticosteroid. J Neuroophthalmol 2006;26:65.

51. Pletcher SD, Sindwani R, Metson R. Endoscopic orbital and optic nerve decompression. Otolaryngol Clin North Am 2006;39:943.

52. Harris GJ. Orbital vascular malformations: a consensus statement on terminology and its clinical implications. Orbital Society. Am J Ophthalmol 1999;127:453.

53. Katowitz J. Pediatric oculoplastic surgery. New York (NY): Springer; 2002.

54. Moretti A, Croce A, Leone O, et al. Osteoma of maxillary sinus: case report. Acta Otorhinolaryngol Ital 2004;24:219.

55. Eller R, Sillers M. Common fibro-osseous lesions of the paranasal sinuses. Otolaryngol Clin North Am 2006;39:585.

Endoscopic Surgery of Pituitary Tumors

Rataphol Chris Dhepnorrarat, MBBS, FRACS[a],
Beng Ti Ang, MBBS, FRCSEd(SN)[b],
Dharambir Singh Sethi, MBBS, FRCSEd[a,*]

KEYWORDS

- Endoscopic skull base surgery • Functional pituitary adenoma
- Secretory pituitary adenoma • Endocrine outcomes

EBM Question	Level of Evidence	Grade of Recommendation
Does endoscopic surgery improve control of functional tumors?	4	C

With rapid advances in technology and endoscopic techniques in the 1980s and early 1990s, endoscopic sinus surgery expanded beyond the realms of the paranasal sinuses and into the skull base. In the early 1990s, endoscopic approaches to the skull base were described. Jankowski and colleagues[1] reported on the endoscopic approach to the sella in 3 patients in 1992. Sethi and Pillay[2] at the Singapore General Hospital reported on a series of 40 patients using an endonasal transsphenoidal technique for the management of sellar lesions. A series of 45 cases of endoscope-assisted pituitary surgery was reported by the Pittsburgh group in 1996,[3] and in 1999, Cappabianca and colleagues[4] reported a series of purely endoscopic approaches to the sella. Many proponents of the endoscopic approach reported superior panoramic vision and improved appreciation of the relationships of the structures surrounding the sella turcica compared with the operating microscope. These advantages facilitated further developments in techniques and reconstruction to allow surgery in structures beyond the sella. The concept of extended approaches to the skull base evolved,[5–8] enabling the endoscopic surgeon to manage larger tumors with suprasellar extension and local invasion.

The authors have nothing to disclose.
[a] Department of Otorhinolaryngology, Singapore General Hospital, Outram Road, Singapore 169608
[b] Department of Neurosurgery, National Neuroscience Institute, 11 Jalan Tan Tock Seng, Singapore 308433
* Corresponding author.
E-mail address: sethi.dharmbir@sgh.com.sg

The ability of endoscopic pituitary surgery to control hormonal dysfunction holds great appeal because it may reduce the risks associated with other surgical approaches and addresses many of the disadvantages of radiotherapy and medical therapy. After the initial reports of successful endoscopic surgery of pituitary tumors, comparative studies emerged, supporting several advantages over the microsurgical approach. These advantages include reduced blood loss[9,10] and analgesia requirements.[9,11] Shorter hospital admissions have also been reported,[10–13] and intraoperative complications were reduced in several reports.[3,9,11]

EPIDEMIOLOGY

Pituitary adenomas are the most common neoplasms of the pituitary gland. These tumors are more common in females and increase in incidence with age. Although rare in children, these adenomas have been reported to be present in almost 30% of the older population,[14] although most are asymptomatic. Pituitary adenomas account for approximately 5% to 15% of symptomatic intracranial tumors. Although most cases are sporadic, a small proportion is related to syndromes such as the multiple endocrine neoplasia type I syndrome, an autosomal dominant syndrome of pituitary adenomas, parathyroid hyperplasia, and pancreatic tumors.

Adenomas that secrete hormone products account for approximately 90% of pituitary adenomas, according to a report from 1995.[15] This number is now likely to be much lower with the widespread use of imaging, which now detects incidental tumors as small as 2 mm in 10% to 20% of the population.[16] Many functional tumors do not produce hormone products in significant quantities to cause clinically manifest endocrinopathy.

PATHOPHYSIOLOGY

Pituitary adenomas are classified according to their secretory hormone products. They are also arbitrarily classified into microadenomas (<10 mm in size) and macroadenomas (≤10 mm) (**Fig. 1**). Secretory hormones include prolactin, growth hormone (GH) (**Fig. 2**), corticotropin, and, rarely, thyrotropin (TSH). With the exception of incidentalomas, secretory adenomas often present as endocrinopathies and are microadenomas at diagnosis. However, nonfunctional tumors usually present as macroadenomas when they are large enough to produce compressive symptoms (see **Fig. 1**).

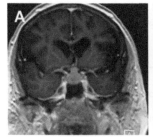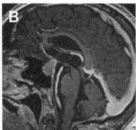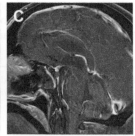

Fig. 1. A small nonfunctioning macroadenoma with early visual field defects. Before (*A*) and after removal (*B*), with a small septal flap used in the reconstruction. The surgical goal differs greatly in the management of this tumor in a 70-year-old man compared with an active GH-secreting adenoma in a 20-year-old man who is not controlled with medical therapy (*C*). (*Courtesy of* Prof Richard Harvey.)

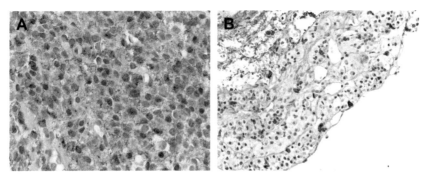

Fig. 2. GH-secreting tumor on histopathology demonstrating background brownish staining (*A*) and compared with normal pituitary (*B*). (*Courtesy of* Prof Richard Harvey and Dr Peter Earls.)

CLINICAL FEATURES
Prolactin-Secreting Adenomas

In women who have not had a recent pregnancy, galactorrhea is the most common endocrinologic sequelae of prolactinomas. This condition may be accompanied by amenorrhea (Forbes-Albright syndrome). Men present with sexual dysfunction, infertility, obesity, and gynecomastia.

ACTH-Secreting Adenomas

In patients who are not treated with steroids, Cushing syndrome (the clinical manifestations of adrenal glucocorticoid hypersecretion) is most commonly caused by a pituitary adenoma. This scenario, termed Cushing disease, is more common in females. Presenting features include weight gain, widening of the face (moon facies), mood alterations, diabetes, and hypertension.

GH-Secreting Adenomas

GH-secreting adenomas present with acromegaly in adults. There is coarseness of facial features with enlargement of hands and feet, along with hirsutism, diabetes, hypertension, and hypertrophic arthropathy. As the dysmorphic features develop gradually over years or decades, patients tend to present with larger tumors than those with other secretory adenomas.

TSH-Secreting Tumors

TSH-secreting tumors account for less than 3% of pituitary adenomas.[17] They present with thyrotoxicosis.

Visual Symptoms

Nonfunctional adenomas tend to present as macroadenomas causing visual symptoms. However, neural compression can also be a feature of functional adenomas. Classically, there is compression of the optic chiasm producing bitemporal visual field deficits. As the adenoma compresses the chiasm from below, the superior bitemporal quadrants tend to be affected more than the inferior quadrants. Long-standing compression of optic axons may lead to reduced visual acuity, and monocular deficits may result from compression of the lateral aspect of the chiasm or compression of only one optic nerve. Ophthalmoplegia may result from cavernous sinus involvement, with the third cranial nerve being the most commonly affected.[18]

Pituitary Apoplexy

Sudden enlargement of a pituitary adenoma resulting from hemorrhage or infarction may result in headache, altered consciousness, and ophthalmoplegia, with or without visual loss. This condition may be fatal and usually has no identifiable precipitants. Known predisposing factors include head trauma, radiation treatment, bromocriptine, pregnancy, surgery, and anticoagulation.[18]

INVESTIGATION

Investigations for pituitary adenomas include a comprehensive visual assessment, hormone analysis, and radiology. These investigations are important to characterize the tumor and to establish a baseline from which the results of treatment can be measured. Secretory tumors may not produce clinical endocrinopathy and are thus diagnosed on biochemical analysis. Prolactin-secreting tumors are diagnosed when serum levels are 10 times more than the normal limit. The level of prolactin is increased during pregnancy and lactation and when a tumor (functional or not) compresses the pituitary stalk and reduces the dopaminergic inhibition of prolactin secretion. Final histopathologic tests can distinguish between hyperplasia and true prolactinomas (**Fig. 3**). High-field magnetic resonance imaging with and without gadolinium is the

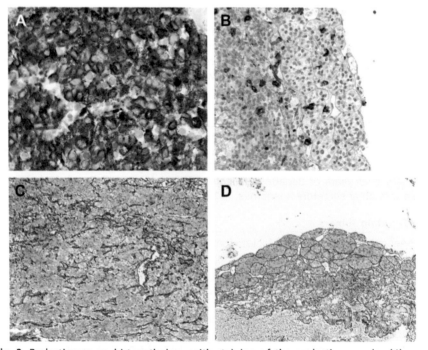

Fig. 3. Prolactinoma on histopathology with staining of the prolactin granules (*A*) compared with normal pituitary (*B*). The reticulin stain demonstrates broken architecture (*C*) in true adenomas compared with hyperplasia (*D*). (*Courtesy of* Prof Richard Harvey and Dr Peter Earls.)

imaging modality of choice, and a computed tomographic scan may be helpful in preoperative planning (**Fig. 4**). Pituitary adenomas often are very large (**Fig. 5**) and display bone erosion (**Fig. 6**).

MANAGEMENT

As well as the control of hormonal secretion, the goals of treatment of pituitary adenomas include decompression of the optic nerve and other neurologic structures by reduction of tumor size, total resection in some cases, and the access to tissue for a histologic diagnosis. Other goals of surgery include minimization of complications from intervention and prevention of disease recurrence. Not all these goals are sufficiently addressed by all treatment modalities, so treatment choices are made by balancing the priorities and the perceived risks and disadvantages (see **Fig. 5**).

Treatment of pituitary adenomas is pursued more vigilantly than many other benign tumors because the location of the pituitary complex predisposes tumors in that region to produce neurologic complications that may not be reversible, particularly visual deficits. Because most adenomas are functional, treatment is necessary for control of hormonal dysfunction (see **Fig. 4**). The risk of pituitary apoplexy adds impetus for treatment.

PROGNOSIS AND NATURAL HISTORY

The natural history of pituitary adenomas is not well understood. Karavitaki and colleagues[19] reported on a series of nonfunctioning tumors observed over an average of 42 months. The investigators found that of the 16 microadenomas and 24 macroadenomas, the 48-month probability of enlargement was 19% for microadenomas and 44% for macroadenomas. Of the tumors that demonstrated growth, 57% had associated deterioration of vision.

ENDOSCOPIC SURGERY VERSUS MICROSURGICAL PROCEDURES

One meta-analysis of short-term outcomes of endoscopic pituitary surgery was compiled in 2009 by Tabaee and colleagues.[20] This report included 8 studies[9–11,13,21–24] as well as the investigators' own series, all of which were published in 2000 or after.

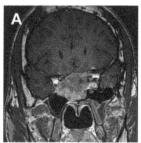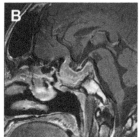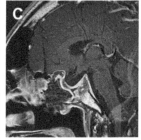

Fig. 4. A GH-secreting tumor after medical therapy in a patient presenting with gigantism. The diaphragm has descended with medical therapy and tumor shrinkage but extensive tumor bulk remains (*A, B*) and the endocrinopathy persists. The resection is often aggressive with an attempt at true tumor resection (cf debulking). The ability to repair cerebrospinal fluid (CSF) leaks reliably with a septal flap shifts the philosophy to aggressive tumor resection in which only cavernous sinus and cranial nerve injury dictates the ability to remove tumor rather than CSF leak concerns (*C*). (*Courtesy of* Prof Richard Harvey.)

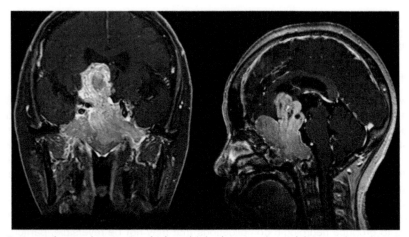

Fig. 5. A very large adenoma in which multiple therapeutic modalities and combination of surgical approaches will be used to manage the neoplasm. The residual disease in this patient will be managed with stereotactic radiotherapy. (*Courtesy of* Prof Richard Harvey.)

Before the release of the consensus statement for the cure of acromegaly,[25] studies did not report on uniform definitions for biochemical control. The meta-analysis revealed a gross tumor removal rate of 78% (95% confidence interval [CI], 67%–89%). Functioning pituitary adenomas accounted for 293 of the total 821 cases. For hormonal control, endoscopic surgery was found to be successful in a high proportion of patients. Hormonal control for 53 ACTH-secreting tumors was 81% (95% CI, 71%–91%), and hormonal remission was seen in 84% (95% CI, 76%–92%) of the 82 GH-secreting tumors and 82% (95% CI, 70%–94%) of the 158 prolactin-secreting tumors. The same meta-analysis pooled the complication rates of the 9 studies and found cerebrospinal fluid leaks in 2% (95% CI, 0%–4%); diabetes insipidus in 6% (95% CI, 4%–9%), including permanent diabetes insipidus in 1% (0%–2%); epistaxis in less than 1% (0%–1%); and anterior pituitary dysfunction in less than 1% (0%–1%). Two deaths were reported from vascular injury (0.24%).

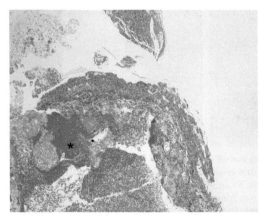

Fig. 6. Aggressive, but not malignant, GH-secreting adenoma invading the bone (*asterisk*). (*Courtesy of* Dr Peter Earls.)

Dorward[26] used the same criteria as the earlier meta-analysis to include a further 12 studies[27–38] in addition to those used in the meta-analysis. Raw data from the 21 studies were used to assess the outcomes of 512 endoscopic procedures for functional pituitary adenomas. The remission rates for GH-secreting, ACTH-secreting, and prolactin-secreting tumors were 69% (138/199), 74% (119/161), and 74% (112/152), respectively. The overall remission rate was 72% (369/512). As expected, the remission rates were higher for microadenomas (84%) than for macroadenomas (69%) or invasive tumors (40%). Dorward[26] also compared the results of the endoscopic series with the results of microsurgical resections of pituitary adenomas, applying the same selection and exclusion criteria. In calculating this comparison, Dorward used the overall weighted rates that were applied in the original meta-analysis by Tabaee. Eight microsurgical studies for acromegaly were included[39–46] along with microsurgical studies for Cushing disease and prolactinomas. The results, displayed in **Table 1**, demonstrate similar remission rates for all the functional adenomas. Comparing the 2 surgical techniques in greater detail revealed a trend for higher remission rates for endoscopic procedures for microadenomas (84% vs 77%). However, there was a marked difference for achieving hormonal remission between the 2 approaches for macroadenomas. Although endocrine remission was seen in 70% of macroadenomas resected endoscopically, it was found in only 45% of microscopic resections. **Table 2** compares the hormone remission rates after surgery for microadenomas and macroadenomas.

Mortini and colleagues[47] retrospectively reviewed an institutional experience with transsphenoidal microsurgical resection of pituitary adenomas. The investigators reported that of a total of 762 patients with functional adenomas, surgery achieved control in 504 (66.1%). Success rates were poorer for macroadenomas (55.5%) than for microadenomas (78.9%) and poorer for tumors involving the cavernous sinus. Although the success rate for macroadenomas was higher than in the microsurgery studies reported by Dorward, it still falls short of the results seen with endoscopic resections (see **Table 2**).

STEREOTACTIC RADIOSURGERY AND RADIOTHERAPY

Several publications exist on the use of stereotactic radiotherapy for active pituitary adenomas. However, a significant amount of variation exists in the literature. Studies vary in their definition of hormonal remission, inclusion and exclusion criteria, and follow-up periods. Most studies also include patients who had surgery before their radiotherapy as well as those who did not, making a comparison between radiotherapy and surgery difficult. Rates of endocrine remission vary greatly, and most series report higher marginal doses used for functioning tumors (typically 20–25 Gy). Starke and colleagues[48] published an evidence-based review of radiotherapy and stereotactic radiosurgery for Cushing disease, including 39 studies with 731 patients. This study revealed rates of tumor growth control of 66% to 100% and endocrine remission rates of 17% to 100%. Because stereotactic radiosurgery is associated with lower rates of complications than traditional methods, it is emerging as the preferred modality of radiotherapy.

Wan and colleagues[49] reported on a series of 347 patients who received Gamma Knife radiosurgery, of whom 47 had prior surgery. Using strict criteria for biochemical cure, normalization of hormone levels was seen in 27.9% of ACTH-secreting adenomas, 23.3% of prolactinomas, and 36.9% for GH-secreting adenomas. These results are substantially inferior to those from surgical techniques, despite a high success rate of radiosurgery for preventing further tumor growth (91.6%). The study

Table 1
Treatment modalities for functional pituitary adenomas and hormone remission rates of selected studies

Study	Treatment	Study Type	Number of Patients with Functional Tumors	Overall Hormone Remission Rate (%)	Cushing Disease Remission Rate (%)	GH Remission Rate (%)	Prolactin Remission Rate (%)
Dorward,[26] 2010	Endoscopic surgery	Meta-analysis of 21 studies	512	75	75	72	78
Doward,[26] 2010	Microsurgical resection	Meta-analysis	NR	73	78	78	62
Mortini et al,[47] 2005	Microsurgical resection	Case series	762	66	77.5	59	62
Wan et al,[49] 2009	Gamma Knife	Case series	347	28	29	27	23
Sheehan et al,[51] 2011	Gamma Knife	Case series	244	NR	54	53	26
Molitch,[52] 2003	Bromocriptine	Review study	997	—	—	—	76
Molitch,[52] 2003	Cabergoline	Review study	612	—	—	—	89
Verhelst et al,[56] 1991	Metyrapone	Case series	53	—	75[a]	—	—
Freda et al,[57] 2005	Octreotide	Meta-analysis	614	—	—	57	—
Cozzi et al,[58] 2006	Octreotide	Prospective series	67	—	—	69	—

Abbreviation: NR, not recorded.
[a] By inhibition of steroidogenesis.

Table 2 Hormone remission rates for surgical treatment of functional pituitary adenomas according to tumor size			
Study	Surgical Technique	Microadenoma Hormone Remission Rate (%)	Macroadenoma Hormone Remission Rate (%)
Dorward,[26] 2010	Endoscopic surgery	84	70
Dorward,[26] 2010	Microscopic resection	77	45
Mortini et al,[47] 2005	Microscopic resection	79	55.5

by Wan and colleagues[49] found that the overall normalization of hormone levels was 28.2%, and a further 61.1% had a decrease in hormone hypersecretion. Complications of treatment seem to be low, with hypopituitarism seen in only 6 (1.7%) patients. This low rate compares favorably with older series using conventional radiotherapy. The investigators confirmed that the effects of radiotherapy may take as long as 3 years to stabilize, representing a distinct disadvantage of this treatment modality, particularly with Cushing disease, in which control of hormone levels is more urgent. The study by Wan and colleagues[49] and other research[50] suggest that the mean time to remission is approximately 1 year.

In a recent large study by Sheehan and colleagues,[51] Gamma Knife radiosurgery was found to achieve hormonal remission rates of 53% for GH-secreting adenomas, 54% for Cushing disease, and 26% for prolactinomas. The median remission times, however, were 29.8 months for GH-secreting tumors, 13.0 months for Cushing disease, and 24.5 months for prolactinomas. The 418 patients included 244 patients with functioning tumors, some of whom had failed prior surgery or medical therapy. New pituitary hormone deficiency, which was seen in 24.4%, was significantly related to large tumor volume, use of pituitary hormone–suppressive therapy, and prior craniotomy. No patients had panhypopituitarism. Partial cranial nerve palsy was present in 5 patients, and 8 patients developed new visual field or acuity defects. Although this study represents the largest published series of patients treated with Gamma Knife radiosurgery, the median follow-up was only 31 months, with some patients having as little as 6 months of follow-up.

MEDICAL THERAPY

Medical treatment is usually satisfactory for patients with prolactinomas. However, control of hormone levels and compressive symptoms is not universal, and the side effects of dopaminergic medications may warrant alternative treatments. In one report, normal hormone levels were achieved in 76% of 997 patients on bromocriptine, 87% of 98 patients on pergolide, and 89% of 612 patients treated with cabergoline.[52] Biller and colleagues[53] reviewed several studies to demonstrate that tumor reduction of at least 50% can be attained when treatment is continued for more than 12 months in 64% of patients treated with bromocriptine, 86% of patients treated with pergolide, and 96% of patients treated with cabergoline. The side effects of dopamine agonists are similar, the most common being nausea and vomiting ($\sim$30%), headache ($\sim$30%), and dizziness ($\sim$25%).[52] Although cabergoline seems to be better tolerated, it is associated with rare cases of cardiac valvular insufficiency, demonstrated in a meta-analysis.[54]

Currently, no medical treatment offers the potential for curing Cushing disease. Adrenal-directed therapy includes inhibition of steroidogenesis (ketoconazole and metyrapone) and direct inhibition of adrenal cortex (mitotane and etomidate). Ketoconazole may normalize the urine-free cortisol levels in 80% of patients but has significant adverse effects, including abnormal liver function test results (15%), gynecomastia (13%), gastrointestinal effects (8%), and rash (2%).[55] Metyrapone has been shown to control hormone levels in 75%, with side effects of hirsutism (70%), dizziness and ataxia (15%), nausea and vomiting (5%), and rash (4%).[56] Pituitary-directed medical treatment of Cushing disease includes targeting the dopamine D_2 receptors. A summary of several small series yielding a total of 23 patients treated with bromocriptine revealed normalization of glucocorticoid levels in 42%.[55] Although several other pituitary-directed medical treatments have been used for Cushing disease, evidence for their use is limited.[53]

For the medical management of acromegaly, somatostatin analogues, such as octreotide, are the first choice for many patients, having largely superseded dopamine agonists.[55] A meta-analysis by Freda and colleagues[57] of neoadjuvant octreotide treatment demonstrated GH levels of less than 2.5 μg/L in 57% and normalization of insulinlike growth factor 1 (IGF-1) levels in 67%. Cozzi and colleagues[58] conducted a prospective study with long-term follow-up using octreotide as a first-line treatment and achieved GH levels less than 2.5 μg/L in 68.7% and normal IGF-1 levels in 70.1%; however, tumor size control is inferior to rates seen in surgical series.

SUMMARY

Although several modalities of treatment exist for the treatment of functional pituitary adenomas, endoscopic pituitary surgery has emerged as the first-line treatment of choice, with the exception of prolactinomas. The rates of hormonal remission and reduction in tumor size are not inferior to any of the other treatment modalities (level 4 evidence). Surgery offers immediate decompression of neurologic structures with a low rate of complications, and there is also potential for immediate control of hormonal function. The delay in improvement seen with radiotherapy is a distinct disadvantage, especially in the setting of deteriorating vision or other neurologic sequelae or for patients with significant morbidity as a result of hormonal imbalance. Medical treatment, in most cases, does not address the underlying cause of disease and requires lifelong therapy. Medical treatment may also be complicated by difficulties with dose titration, administration, and adverse effects. Although reliable long-term data are lacking, a substantial rate of hormonal dysfunction after a period of remission is seen in patients treated with surgery and radiotherapy. Therefore, all patients should have long-term follow-up after treatment.

Comparisons of endoscopic and microscopic techniques have demonstrated the advantages of endoscopic surgery, particularly for macroadenomas (level 4 evidence). The use of angled endoscopes improves the visual field at the operating site and hence facilitates more complete tumor removal. Also, by avoiding the use of the microscope, the view of the surgeon is less inhibited by the presence of instruments. These are likely to be factors contributing to the superior results seen with macroadenomas. Endoscopic resections are also associated with shorter recovery times and reduced complications.

EBM Question	Author's reply
Does endoscopic surgery improve control of functional tumors?	Rates of hormonal remission and tumour control are similar to microscopic and open techniques but with less perioperative morbidity.

REFERENCES

1. Jankowski RD, Auque J, Simon C, et al. Endoscopic pituitary tumor surgery. Laryngoscope 1992;102(2):198–202.
2. Sethi DS, Pillay PK. Endoscopic management of lesions of the sella turcica. J Laryngol Otol 1995;109(10):956–62.
3. Jho HD, Carrau RL. Endoscope assisted transsphenoidal surgery for pituitary adenoma. Acta Neurochir 1996;138(12):1416–25.
4. Cappabianca P, Alfieri A, de Divitiis E. Endoscopic endonasal transsphenoidal approach to the sella: towards functional endoscopic pituitary surgery (FEPS). Minim Invasive Neurosurg 1998;41(2):66–73.
5. Kaptain GJ, Vincent DA, Sheehan JP, et al. Transsphenoidal approaches for the extracapsular resection of midline suprasellar and anterior cranial base lesions. Neurosurgery 2001;49(1):94–101.
6. Jho HD, Ha HG. Endoscopic endonasal skull base surgery: part 1—the midline anterior fossa skull base. Minim Invasive Neurosurg 2004;47(1):1–8.
7. Jho HD, Ha HG. Endoscopic endonasal skull base surgery: part 2—the cavernous sinus. Minim Invasive Neurosurg 2004;47(1):9–15.
8. Jho HD, Ha HG. Endoscopic endonasal skull base surgery: part 3—the clivus and posterior fossa. Minim Invasive Neurosurg 2004;47(1):16–23.
9. Casler JD, Doolittle AM, Mair EA. Endoscopic surgery of the anterior skull base. Laryngoscope 2005;115(1):16–24.
10. White DR, Sonnenburg RE, Ewend MG, et al. Safety of minimally invasive pituitary surgery (MIPS) compared with a traditional approach. Laryngoscope 2004; 114(11):1945–8.
11. Cho DY, Liau WR. Comparison of endonasal endoscopic surgery and sublabial microsurgery for prolactinomas. Surg Neurol 2002;58(6):371–5.
12. Cappabianca P, Cavallo LM, Colao A, et al. Endoscopic endonasal transsphenoidal approach: outcome analysis of 100 consecutive procedures. Minim Invasive Neurosurg 2002;45(4):193–200.
13. Jho HD. Endoscopic transsphenoidal surgery. J Neurooncol 2001;54(2):187–95.
14. Gold EB. Epidemiology of pituitary tumors. Epidemiol Rev 1981;3:163–83.
15. Aron DC, Tyrrell JB, Wilson CB. Pituitary tumors; current concepts in diagnosis and management. West J Med 1995;162(4):340–52.
16. Aron DC, Howlett TA. Pituitary incidentalomas. Endocrinol Metab Clin North Am 2000;29(1):205–21.
17. Mindermann T, Wilson CB. Thyrotropin-producing pituitary adenomas. J Neurosurg 1993;79(4):521–7.
18. Gittinger JW Jr. Pituitary tumors. In: Miller NR, Newman NJ, Biousse V, et al, editors. Walsh & Hoyt's clinical neuro-ophthalmology. 6th edition. Philadelphia: Lippincott Williams & Wilkins; 2005. p. 1532–46.
19. Karavitaki N, Collison K, Halliday J, et al. What is the natural history of non-operated nonfunctional pituitary adenomas? Clin Endocrinol (Oxf) 2007;67(6): 938–43.
20. Tabaee A, Anand VK, Barrón Y, et al. Endoscopic pituitary surgery: a systematic review and meta-analysis. J Neurosurg 2009;111(3):545–54.
21. Cappabianca P, Cavallo LM, Colao A, et al. Surgical complications associated with the endoscopic endonasal transsphenoidal approach for pituitary adenomas. J Neurosurg 2002;97(2):293–8.
22. Kabil MS, Eby JB, Shahinian HK. Fully endoscopic endonasal vs. transseptal transsphenoidal pituitary surgery. Minim Invasive Neurosurg 2005;48(6):348–54.

23. Rudnik A, Zawadzki T, Wojtacha M, et al. Endoscopic transnasal transsphenoidal treatment of pathology of the sellar region. Minim Invasive Neurosurg 2005;48(2): 101–7.
24. Shen CC, Wang YC, Hua WS, et al. Endoscopic endonasal transsphenoidal surgery for pituitary tumors. Chin Med J (Engl) 2000;63(4):301–10.
25. Giustina A, Barkan A, Casanueva FF, et al. Criteria for cure of acromegaly: a consensus statement. J Clin Endocrinol Metab 2000;85(2):526–9.
26. Dorward N. Endocrine outcomes in endoscopic pituitary surgery: a literature review. Acta Neurochir 2010;152(8):1275–9.
27. Charalampaki P, Ayyad A, Kockro RA, et al. Surgical complications after endoscopic transsphenoidal pituitary surgery. J Clin Neurosci 2009;16(6):786–9.
28. Choe JH, Lee KS, Jeun SS, et al. Endocrine outcome of endoscopic endonasal transsphenoidal surgery in functioning pituitary adenomas. J Korean Neurosurg Soc 2008;44(3):151–5.
29. Dehdashti AR, Ganna A, Karabatsou K, et al. Pure endoscopic endonasal approach for pituitary adenomas: early surgical results in 200 patients and comparison with previous microsurgical series. Neurosurgery 2008;62(5):1006–17.
30. D'Haens J, Van Rompaey K, Stadnik T, et al. Fully endoscopic transsphenoidal surgery for functioning pituitary adenomas: a retrospective comparison with traditional transsphenoidal microsurgery in the same institution. Surg Neurol 2009; 72(4):336–40.
31. Frank G, Pasquini E, Farneti G, et al. The endoscopic versus the traditional approach in pituitary surgery. Neuroendocrinology 2006;83(3–4):240–8.
32. Gondim JA, Schops M, de Almeida JP, et al. Endoscopic endonasal transsphenoidal surgery: surgical results of 228 pituitary adenomas treated in a pituitary center. Pituitary 2010;13(1):68–77.
33. Koc K, Anik I, Ozdamar D, et al. The learning curve in endoscopic pituitary surgery and our experience. Neurosurg Rev 2006;29(4):298–305.
34. Netea-Maier RT, van Lindert EJ, den Heijer M, et al. Transsphenoidal pituitary surgery via the endoscopic technique: results in 35 consecutive patients with Cushing's disease. Eur J Endocrinol 2006;154(5):675–84.
35. Rudnik A, Kos-Kudła B, Larysz D, et al. Endoscopic transsphenoidal treatment of hormonally active pituitary adenomas. Neuro Endocrinol Lett 2007;28(4): 438–44.
36. Shah S, Har-El G. Diabetes insipidus after pituitary surgery: incidence after traditional versus endoscopic transsphenoidal approaches. Am J Rhinol 2001;15(6): 377–9.
37. Uren B, Vrodos N, Wormald PJ. Fully endoscopic transsphenoidal resection of pituitary tumors: technique and results. Am J Rhinol 2007;21(4):510–4.
38. Zhang Y, Wang Z, Liu Y, et al. Endoscopic transsphenoidal treatment of pituitary adenomas. Neurol Res 2008;30:581–6.
39. Abe T, Lüdecke DK. Effects of preoperative octreotide treatment on different subtypes of 90 GH-secreting pituitary adenomas and outcome in one surgical centre. Eur J Endocrinol 2001;145(2):137–45.
40. Beauregard C, Truong U, Hardy J, et al. Long-term outcome and mortality after transsphenoidal adenomectomy for acromegaly. Clin Endocrinol 2003;58(1):86–91.
41. De P, Rees DA, Davies N, et al. Transsphenoidal surgery for acromegaly in Wales: results based on stringent criteria of remission. J Clin Endocrinol Metab 2003; 88(8):3567–72.
42. Kaltsas GA, Isidori AM, Florakis D, et al. Predictors of the outcome of surgical treatment in acromegaly and the value of the mean growth hormone day curve

in assessing postoperative disease activity. J Clin Endocrinol Metab 2001;86(4): 1645–52.

43. Laws ER, Vance ML, Thapar K. Pituitary surgery for the management of acromegaly. Horm Res 2000;53(Suppl 3):71–5.

44. Nomikos P, Buchfelder M, Fahlbusch R. The outcome of surgery in 668 patients with acromegaly using current criteria of biochemical 'cure'. Eur J Endocrinol 2005;152(3):379–87.

45. Shimon I, Cohen ZR, Ram Z, et al. Transsphenoidal surgery for acromegaly: endocrinological follow-up of 98 patients. Neurosurgery 2001;48(6):1239–43.

46. Trepp R, Stettler C, Zwahlen M, et al. Treatment outcomes and mortality of 94 patients with acromegaly. Acta Neurochir 2005;147(3):243–51.

47. Mortini P, Losa M, Barzaghi R, et al. Results of transsphenoidal surgery in a large series of patients with pituitary adenoma. Neurosurgery 2005;56(6):1222–33.

48. Starke RM, Williams BJ, Vance ML, et al. Radiation therapy and stereotactic radiosurgery for the treatment of Cushing's disease: an evidence-based review. Curr Opin Endocrinol Diabetes Obes 2010;17(4):356–64.

49. Wan H, Chihiro O, Yuan S. MASEP gamma knife for secretory pituitary adenomas: experience in 347 consecutive cases. J Exp Clin Cancer Res 2009;28(1):36.

50. Laws E, Vance ML. Radiosurgery for pituitary tumors and craniopharyngiomas. Neurosurg Clin N Am 1999;10(2):327–36.

51. Sheehan JP, Pouratian N, Steiner L, et al. Gamma Knife surgery for pituitary adenomas: factors related to radiological and endocrine outcomes. J Neurosurg 2011;114(2):303–9.

52. Molitch ME. Dopamine resistance of prolactinomas. Pituitary 2003;6(1):19–27.

53. Biller BM, Calao A, Petersenn S, et al. Prolactinomas, Cushing's disease and acromegaly: debating the role of medical therapy for secretory pituitary adenomas. BMC Endocr Disord 2010;10:10.

54. Bogazzi F, Manetti L, Raffaelli V, et al. Cabergoline therapy and the risk of cardiac valve regurgitation in patients with hyperprolactinemia: a meta-analysis from clinical studies. J Endocrinol Invest 2008;31(12):1119–23.

55. Miller JW, Crapo L. The medical treatment of Cushing's syndrome. Endocr Rev 1993;14(4):443–58.

56. Verhelst JA, Trainer PJ, Howlett TA, et al. Short and long-term responses to metyrapone in the medical management of 91 patients with Cushing's syndrome. Clin Endocrinol (Oxf) 1991;35(2):169–78.

57. Freda PU, Katznelson L, van der Lely AJ, et al. Long-acting somatostatin analog therapy of acromegaly: a meta-analysis. J Clin Endocrinol Metab 2005;90(8): 4465–73.

58. Cozzi R, Montini M, Attanasio R, et al. Primary treatment of acromegaly with octreotide LAR: a long-term (up to 9 years) prospective study of its efficacy in the control of disease activity and tumor shrinkage. J Clin Endocrinol Metab 2006; 91(4):1397–403.

Craniopharyngioma

Aldo C. Stamm, MD, PhD[a], Eduardo Vellutini, MD, PhD[b],
Leonardo Balsalobre, MD[a,c],*

KEYWORDS

• Craniopharyngioma • Endoscopic • Endonasal • Outcomes

EBM Question	Level of Evidence	Grade of Recommendation
Is morbidity decreased in patients with endoscopic resection of craniopharyngiomas (vision, pituitary function) compared to microscopic/trans-cranial surgery?	4	C

Craniopharyngiomas are rare epithelial-squamous, extra-axial tumors arising along the path of the craniopharyngeal duct, with slow-growing characteristic. Two hypotheses explain the origin of craniopharyngioma—embryogenetic and metaplastic; they complement each other and explain the craniopharyngioma spectrum.[1]

EPIDEMIOLOGY

The overall incidence of craniopharyngioma is approximately 0.5 to 2 per 100,000 per year. The Central Brain Tumor Registry of the United States revealed an average of 338 cases diagnosed annually, with 96 occurring in children aged 0 to 4 years in this country. No variance by gender or race was found.[2] The age distribution is bimodal with a peak in childhood and a second peak among middle-aged and older adults.[3] No definite genetic relationship has been found and few familial cases reported.[1]

PATHOPHYSIOLOGY

There are 2 hypotheses to justify the craniopharyngioma spectrum: embryogenetic (neoplastic transformation of embryonic squamous cell rests of the involuted

The authors have nothing to disclose.
[a] São Paulo ENT Center, Professor Edmundo Vasconcelos Hospital, Rua Afonso Braz, 525, conj. 13. Vila Nova Conceição. CEP: 04511-011, São Paulo, Brazil
[b] DFV Neurosurgery, Rua Adma Jafet, 74 cj.121. CEP: 01308-050, São Paulo, Brazil
[c] Department of Otolaryngology, Federal University of São Paulo, Rua Afonso Braz, 525, conj. 13. Vila Nova Conceição. CEP: 04511-011, São Paulo, Brazil
* Corresponding author. Rua Afonso Brás, 525, conj. 13. Vila Nova Conceição. CEP: 04511-011, São Paulo, São Paulo, Brazil.
E-mail address: leo_balsalobre@uol.com.br

Otolaryngol Clin N Am 44 (2011) 937–952
doi:10.1016/j.otc.2011.06.015
0030-6665/11/$ – see front matter © 2011 Elsevier Inc. All rights reserved.

craniopharyngeal duct) and metaplastic (metaplasia of adenohypophyseal cells in the pituitary stalk or gland).

Designated as World Health Organization grade I tumors, comprising 2% to 5% of all central nervous system tumors,[4] craniopharyngiomas can be classified in 2 histologic subtypes: adamantinomatous and papillary. The adamantinomatous type may be encountered at any age but predominantly in the first 2 decades of life. The papillary variety has been primarily reported in adults.[5] Some investigators report a lower recurrence rate with the papillary variety, whereas others have found no difference in surgical outcome or recurrence between the 2 subtypes.[5,6]

Craniopharyngiomas are dysontogenic tumors with benign histology and malignant behavior with infiltrative tendency into critical parasellar structures, such as optic apparatus, pituitary stalk and gland, floor of the third ventricle, hypothalamus, and cerebral vasculature of the circle of Willis, and recur after what was thought to be total resection.[7]

The tumor characteristics are solid (with or without calcification) and cystic. The cyst is filled with a turbid, proteinaceous material of brownish-yellow color that glitters and sparkles because of a high content of floating cholesterol crystals. Because of its appearance, it has been compared with machinery oil.[1]

It occur most often in sellar/suprasellar region but can have anterior extension to the prechiasmatic cistern and subfrontal spaces; posterior extension into the prepontine and interpeduncular cisterns, cerebellopontine angle, third ventricle, posterior fossa, and foramen magnum; and laterally toward the subtemporal spaces. They can even reach the sylvian fissure.

Craniopharyngiomas are supplied with blood coming from the anterior circulation: perforators from anterior cerebral artery and the proximal portion of the posterior communicating artery.

Tumor adhesion is the result of local inflammation. Several inflammatory cytokines have been shown to be elevated in the craniopharyngioma cyst fluid compared with cerebrospinal fluid (CSF).[1]

Clinical

Craniopharyngiomas are highly complex benign tumors and they have variable clinical presentation, the severity of which depends on the location, size, and growth potential of the tumor.[7] Neurologic symptoms may include headaches, nausea, and vomiting. Childhood populations can present, more commonly than adults, hydrocephalus in 41% to 54% of cases.[7] Because of the proximity to the optic chiasm, visual field defects usually present as bitemporal hemianopia, reported in as many as 49% of cases.[8,9]

Pituitary symptoms are associated with growth failure and delayed puberty (in children) and hypogonadism in adults. Rates for pituitary hormone deficits include 35% to 95% for growth hormone, 38% to 82% for follicle-stimulating hormone/luteinizing hormone, 21% to 62% for corticotropin (eg, orthostatic hypotension, hypoglycemia, hyperkalemia, cardiac arrhythmias, lethargy, confusion, anorexia, nausea, and vomiting), 21% to 42% for thyroid-stimulating hormone (eg, weight gain, fatigue, cold intolerance, and constipation), and 6% to 38% for antidiuretic hormone.[7]

Three major clinical syndromes have been described and relate to the anatomic location of the craniopharyngioma: a prechiasmal localization typically results in associated findings of optic atrophy (eg, progressive decline of visual acuity and constriction of visual fields); a retrochiasmal location commonly is associated with hydrocephalus, with signs of increased intracranial pressure (eg, papilledema and horizontal double vision); and intrasellar craniopharyngioma usually manifests with headache and endocrinopathy.[1]

Investigation

The diagnostic evaluation for craniopharyngioma includes precontrast and postcontrast CT scans and MRI and, occasionally, cerebral angiography in addition to complete endocrinologic evaluation (baseline serum electrolytes, serum and urine osmolality, thyroid studies, and morning and evening cortisol levels, growth hormone levels, and luteinizing hormone and follicle-stimulating hormone levels, in adolescent and adult patients) and neuro-ophthalmologic evaluation with formal visual field documentation as well as neuropsychological assessment.[1]

Imaging studies strongly suggest the diagnosis: on plain skull radiograph, tumor calcifications can be observed and may also show an abnormal sella (widening of its outlet, uniform expansion, and shortening or erosion of the dorsum sellae).[7]

CT is the ideal modality for the evaluation of the bony anatomy and detection of calcifications of the tumor. MRI is particularly useful for the topographic and structural analysis of the tumor[10] and is the most important imaging modality used to plan the surgical approach, showing the relationship between the tumor and the vascular structures and the optic apparatus.

Management

Surgical excision, with or without adjuvant conventional external beam irradiation, is the primary option to treatment of craniopharyngiomas. Complete resection remains the goal of primary surgery; however, even with the advent of modern surgical techniques, this may not be warranted if it is associated with significant morbidity.[11]

Matson and Crigler, in 1969, postulated that "recurrence of symptoms has been so relentless and rapid in such a high percentage of cases if the tumor is not radically removed, that our conviction becomes steadily stronger that optimum treatment consists in making every effort to affect total excision at the first operation."[12] Total excision must be attempted at the first operation.

The classical operative technique for craniopharyngioma resection is based on various craniotomy approaches (pterional, bifrontal, and interhemispheric); the transsphenoidal route has always been reserved for resection of purely intrasellar masses. In the 1990s, some investigators began recommending the use of extended transsphenoidal approaches for sellar and suprasellar tumors.[13] Due to the difficulty of visualizing structures of interest and the risk of CSF leak, however, this method did not gain wider acceptance. With the evolution of endoscopic surgery and the possibility of improved visualization, several investigators have since reintroduced the extended transsphenoidal approach as an option for resection of intrasellar and suprasellar craniopharyngiomas, with outcomes similar to those provided by traditional approaches. The lower incidence of CSF leak made possible by the use of vascularized flaps played a decisive role in expanding indications for this approach. In light of the complexity of craniopharyngiomas as a disease entity, any method that may increase the possibility of total resection and minimize operative mortality warrants consideration.

Since the work of Wang and colleagues,[14] craniopharyngiomas were defined as midline lesions arising along the pituitary stalk and were classified by level of origin as infradiaphragmatic or supradiaphragmatic. Postsurgical outcomes in patients with supradiaphragmatic craniopharyngiomas are markedly worse than those achieved in patients with infradiaphragmatic tumors.[3,15,16]

Prognosis

The definition of gross total removal (GTR) is the neurosurgeon's intraoperative impression confirmed by the objective measure of a 3-months' postoperative MRI.

Approximately 10% of totally resected craniopharyngiomas recur and the extent of resection is the most significant predictor for recurrence.[17]

Fahlbusch and colleagues[3] showed 86.9% of recurrence-free survival at 5 years and 81.3% at 10 years. In contrast, the rate of recurrence-free survival was 48.8% for subtotal removal (STR) (ie, minor residual tumor) and only 15.6% for partial removal at 10 years of follow-up.

The Sao Paulo experience

After obtaining institutional review board approval, the authors included 18 patients treated with a purely endoscopic approach to craniopharyngiomas, confirmed with histopathological diagnosis.

All patients underwent MRI and CT to classify the tumor. The vertical extension and position relative to the optic chiasm were analyzed. Neurologic, endocrinological and ophthalmologic evaluations, including formal visual field testing, were performed in patients before and after surgery.

The degree of resection was determined by a combination of the intraoperative assessment and 3-month postoperative MRI studies. Resections were considered GTR only if the surgical impression and MRI assessment revealed no residual tumor. Resections were categorized as near total removal (NTR) if more than 95% of the tumor was removed. An STR was considered when more than 70% of the tumor was resected.[18] Finally, a partial resection was indicated when more than 50% of the tumor remained.[12]

Surgery

In the majority of cases, a modified transseptal/transnasal binostril technique was used (described by Stamm).[19]

After topical vasoconstriction with adrenalin applied on cottonoids, local infiltration of the nasal septum mucosa is performed with lidocaine with adrenaline 1:100,000. A nasal septal hemitransfixion incision is performed unilaterally, usually on the right side. The posterior part of the bony septum is removed, leaving the inferior portion as a midline landmark and the sphenoid face exposed. A nasoseptal flap is created on the contralateral side to the hemitransfixion incision. The superior horizontal incision is made 1 cm below the superior aspect of the nasal septum and continued posteriorly across the sphenoid face at the level of the inferior aspect of the sphenoid ostium. The inferior horizontal incision is performed 0.5 cm above the level of the floor of the nose or laterally in the inferior meatus of a larger flap is required. The position of the anterior incision depends on the length required and may be as far forward as the mucocutaneous junction.

After flap harvest, it is placed into the nasopharynx or maxillary sinus until the extirpate phase of the surgery is complete (**Fig. 1**).

The approach is expanded as required by removal of middle and superior turbinates and opening of the maxillary and ethmoid sinus; in cases requiring bilateral exposure anterior to the sphenoid face, partial septectomy is performed.

Commencing at the sphenoid ostium, the maximum amount of the front wall is then removed.

The mucosa of the posterior sphenoid wall is then displaced laterally. Drilling of the thick tuberculum sellae bone and the sella is then performed. An area the entire intercarotid width is thinned down to eggshell thickness with a high-speed drill and then removed. A Kerrison rongeur may be used for additional bone removal. Bone removal much wider and higher than the area exposed in standard pituitary surgery. Bone removal continues along the sphenoid planum (**Fig. 2**). The superior intercavernous sinus is then coagulated with help of a bipolar cautery (**Fig. 3**). The dura is opened above and below the superior intercavernous sinus, exposing the sellar and suprasellar region.

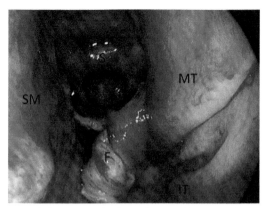

Fig. 1. Endoscopic view of the approach: the right septal mucosa (SM) is preserved. Flap (F) in nasopharynx and the exposure of the sella turcica (S). IT, left inferior turbinate; MT, left middle turbinate.

The intradural resection is performed at first with a debulking of the tumor. Modified transseptal/transnasal binostril approach allows 4 hands; extracapsular sharp dissection and countertraction using gentle suction form the foundation of the endoscopic surgery as they did when microsurgery was performed.

A final inspection is done with a 0° and/or 45° endoscope to identify all the structures, such as pituitary stalk, optic nerves and chiasm, and other cranial nerves and vessels (**Fig. 4**).

Reconstruction

A reliable skull base reconstruction is mandatory at the end of the procedure because of the large dural opening, extensive dissection of arachnoid cisterns and/or third ventricle, and associated CSF leak.[11]

In the beginning of the sao paulo experience, some multilayer free grafts, including fascia lata, fat, and DuraGen (Integra LifeSciences Corp), were used.

At the end of these cases, the authors prefer the triple-F reconstruction (fat, fascia, and flap), with free fat grafts used to fill dead space and form a buttress for a fascia lata inlay graft and, finally, covered with the pedicled nasosseptal flap.

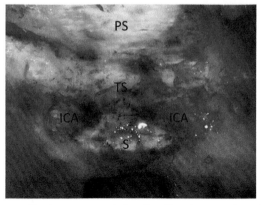

Fig. 2. Dural exposure after bone removal showing the planum sphenoidale (PS), tuberculum sellae (TS), sella turcica (S), and bilateral internal carotid protuberance (ICA).

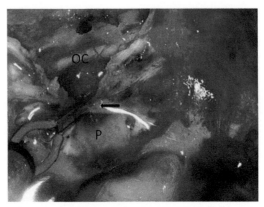

Fig. 3. Bipolar coagulation of superior intercavernous sinus (*arrow*). OC, optic quiasm; P, pituitary gland after dural opening.

Spongostan powder (Ethicon, NJ, USA) and Gelfoam™ (Pfizer, NY, USA) are layered directly over the flap, followed by gauze packing. The packing is supported by a RapidRhino 900 (Arthrocare, Austin, TX, USA) or similar pack.

Postoperative care
Antibiotics are used perioperatively and continued postoperatively while nasal packing remains in situ. Packing is left in place for 5 to 7 days. The onset of diabetes insipidus (DI) is monitored with serum and urine sodium/osmolality measurements. Patients are confined to bed for 48 hours, have 30° head elevation, and avoid straining, Valsalva maneuvers, and nose blowing. Lumbar drains are not routinely used unless there is an additional comorbidity, such as raised intracranial hypertension or prior radiotherapy.

Discharge usually occurs 3 to 5 days postoperatively.

Follow-up
An MRI is performed at 3 months as a baseline study. This is important, because post-surgical MRI signaling is often difficult to interpret. Endocrine assessment is

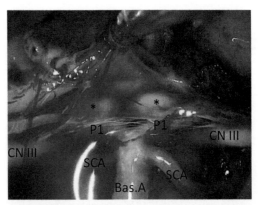

Fig. 4. Zero-degree endoscope inspection after tumor removal. This photo shows basilar artery (Bas. A), superior cerebellar artery (SCA), third cranial nerve (CN III), first segment of posterior cerebral artery (P1), and the mammilary bodies (*asterisk*).

performed routinely in follow-up; however, ophthalmologic evaluation is undertaken only if clinically indicated. The long-term follow-up is multidisciplinary but an endocrinologist is the central team member who coordinates ongoing care.

Results

No patient of the 18 was excluded or lost in follow-up (**Table 1**). There were 11 men and 7 women. Patients' ages ranged from 6 to 72 years (mean age 29.4 years). Seven patients (39%) were under 16 years old, classified as child/young, and 11 (61%) were adults (see **Table 1**).

Two patients (11%) had undergone previous surgery: one had 3 neuroendoscopic procedures, 2 craniotomies and 1 ventricular shunt and the other one had 6 previous procedures: 3 prior craniotomies and 3 radiosurgery.

Clinical presentation

The main symptom presented by patients, visual loss, was observed in 14 of 18 patients (78%). Four of these patients (22%) suffered from panhypopituitarism

Table 1
Signs and symptoms of the 18 patients of the series

Case	Sex	Age (Years)	Anterior Pituitary Function	Posterior Pituitary Function	Visual Function	Previous Treatment
1	M	8	Growth failure	Normal	Normal	None
2	M	15	Panhypopituitarism	DI	Normal	None
3	M	34	Normal	Normal	Visual loss	None
4	F	26	Normal	Normal	Visual loss	None
5	F	7	Normal	DI	Visual loss	None
6	M	36	Panhypopituitarism	Normal	Visual loss	None
7	M	16	Panhypopituitarism	DI	Visual loss	1 VP shunt, 3 neuroendoscopies, and 2 craniotomies
8	F	20	Panhypopituitarism	DI	Visual loss	3 Craniotomy and 3 radiosurgeries
9	M	69	Normal	Normal	Visual loss	None
10	M	24	Normal	Normal	Visual loss	None
11	F	72	Normal	Normal	Visual loss	None
12	M	48	Normal	Normal	Visual loss	None
13	M	29	Hypogonadism	Normal	Visual loss	None
14	F	42	Normal	Normal	Visual loss	None
15	M	09	Growth failure	Normal	Visual loss	None
16	F	06	Growth failure	Normal	Visual loss	None
17	F	12	Growth failure Hypothyroidism	Normal	Normal	None
18	M	56	Hypogonadism Others: cognitive deficits/Somnolence	Normal	Normal	None

Abbreviation: VP shunt, ventriculoperitoneal shunt.

(anterior gland). Three of these 4 patients had DI associated and 1 patient had isolated posterior pituitary function impaired with DI. Two patients (11%) presented with hypogonadism.

Growth failure with somatotrophin deficiency (low insulinlike growth factor 1 levels) was presented alone as first endocrinology presentation in 3 patients. One patient had growth failure and hypothyroidism associated.

In the child/young group, the rate of growth failure with or without other pituitary dysfunction was 85.7% (6 of 7 patients).

One patient was diagnosed in investigation of cognitive deficits with somnolence.

Visual outcomes

Before and after surgery, the patients underwent an ophthalmologic examination, including visual field examination.

Of the 14 patients with preoperative visual deficits, 12 had their vision normalized (**Fig. 5**) or improved (**Fig. 6**), showing a substantial improvement of visual defect rate of 85.7%. One patient's deficit remained stable and another patient had his right vision improved but showed no changes in the left eye (**Table 2**).

Of the 4 patients without preoperative visual deficits, the conditions of 3 patients were unchanged postoperatively, but 1 patient had visual worsening.

Endocrine outcomes

Only 1 of the 4 patients who had preoperative DI improved (case 2), whereas the other 3 remained with deficit (**Table 3**). Nine of the 14 (64%) patients who had normal preoperative function of posterior pituitary experienced new persistent DI after surgery.

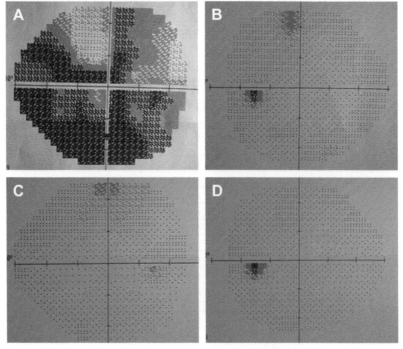

Fig. 5. Visual field test. (*A, B*) preoperative study demonstrating a dense defect, mainly in the right eye. (*C, D*) Postoperative testing showing resolution of visual deficit.

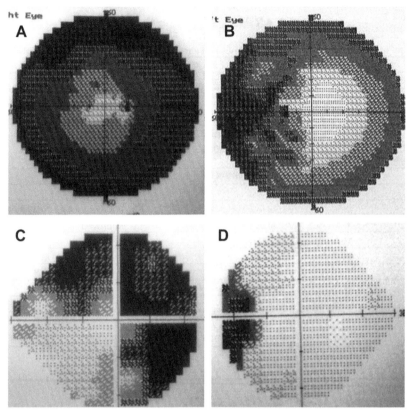

Fig. 6. Visual field test. (*A, B*) Preoperative examination showing an important visual deficits, greatest in the right eye. (*C, D*) Postoperative showing a significant improvement of visual deficit.

None of the 4 patients who had panhypopituitarism improved this condition postoperatively. Of the 14 patients without preoperative panhypopituitarism, 7 (50%) developed panhypopituitarism after the surgery. One patient who had preoperative growth failure experienced the maintenance of this deficit and a new hypothyroidism (case 1). The normalization of an anterior pituitary deficiency after surgery occurred in none of the patients.

Tumor location, surgical approach, and reconstruction
The authors classify tumors based on the location according to the sellar diaphragm as subdiaphragmatic or supradiaphragmatic. The subdiaphragmatic tumors are classified as sellar and/or suprasellar depending on its vertical extension. The supradiaphragmatic are classified as prechiasmatic or postchiasmatic, with or without intraventricular extension.

Five tumors had subdiaphragmatic origin; 4 of these had sellar and suprassellar presentation, and 1 was confined to the sella. In all these cases, the authors used a transsellar approach without the opening of the planum sphenoidale (**Table 4**).

Thirteen tumors had supradiaphragmatic extension, 4 of which were prechiasmatic (**Fig. 7**) and 9 had their location behind the optic chiasm (postchiasmatic) extending into the third ventricle. These tumors were accessed by a transsellar/transplanum

Table 2
Ophthalmologic outcomes

Case	Sex	Preoperative Visual Function	Postoperative Visual Result
1	M	Normal	Remained normal
2	M	Normal	Remained normal
3	M	Visual loss	Improved
4	F	Visual loss	Improved
5	F	Visual loss	Improved right eye
6	M	Visual loss	No improved
7	M	Visual loss	Improved
8	F	Visual loss	Improved
9	M	Visual loss	Improved
10	M	Visual loss	Improved
11	F	Visual loss	Improved
12	M	Visual loss	Improved
13	M	Visual loss	Improved
14	F	Visual loss	Improved
15	M	Visual loss	Improved
16	F	Visual loss	Improved
17	F	Normal	Remained normal
18	M	Normal	Decreased

Table 3
Endocrine outcomes

Case	Anterior Pituitary Function		Posterior Pituitary Function	
	Preoperative	Postoperative	Preoperative	Postoperative
1	Growth failure	Hypothyroidism growth failure	Normal	Normal
2	Panhypopituitarism	Panhypopituitarism	DI	Improved
3	Normal	Normal	Normal	Normal
4	Normal	Normal	Normal	Normal
5	Normal	Normal	DI	DI
6	Panhypopituitarism	Panhypopituitarism	Normal	New DI
7	Panhypopituitarism	Panhypopituitarism	DI	DI
8	Panhypopituitarism	Panhypopituitarism	DI	DI
9	Normal	Normal	Normal	New DI
10	Normal	Normal	Normal	New DI
11	Normal	Panhypopituitarism	Normal	New DI
12	Normal	Normal	Normal	Normal
13	Hypogonadism	Panhypopituitarism	Normal	Normal
14	Normal	Panhypopituitarism	Normal	New DI
15	Growth failure	Panhypopituitarism	Normal	New DI
16	Growth failure	Panhypopituitarism	Normal	New DI
17	Growth failure Hypothyroidism	Panhypopituitarism	Normal	New DI
18	Hypogonadism	Panhypopituitarism	Normal	New DI

Table 4
Tumor characteristics and surgical outcomes

Case	Tumor Location	Surgical Approach	Tumor Removal	Skull Base Reconstruction
1	Subdiaphragmatic (sellar/suprasselar)	Transellar	GTR	Free graft
2	Subdiaphragmatic (sellar/suprasselar)	Transellar	GTR	Free graft
3	Subdiaphragmatic (sellar)	Transellar	GTR	Free graft
4	Subdiaphragmatic (sellar/suprasselar)	Transellar	GTR	Free graft
5	Supradiaphragmatic prechiasmatic	Transellar/transplanum	NTR	Free graft
6	Supradiaphragmatic postchiasmatic—IV	Transellar/transplanum	GTR	3F
7	Supradiaphragmatic postchiasmatic—IV	Transellar/transplanum	NTR	3F
8	Supradiaphragmatic prechiasmatic	Transellar/transplanum	GTR	3F
9	Supradiaphragmatic postchiasmatic—IV	Transellar/transplanum	Partial	3F
10	Supradiaphragmatic postchiasmatic—IV	Transellar/transplanum	STR	3F
11	Supradiaphragmatic postchiasmatic—IV	Transellar/transplanum	STR	3F
12	Supradiaphragmatic prechiasmatic	Transellar/transplanum	NTR	3F
13	Supradiaphragmatic prechiasmatic	Transellar/transplanum	GTR	3F
14	Supradiaphragmatic postchiasmatic—IV	Transellar/transplanum	GTR	3F
15	Subdiaphragmatic (sellar/suprasselar)	Transellar	GTR	3F
16	Supradiaphragmatic postchiasmatic—IV	Transellar/transplanum	GTR	3F
17	Supradiaphragmatic postchiasmatic—IV	Transellar/transplanum	GTR	3F
18	Supradiaphragmatic postchiasmatic—IV	Transellar/transplanum	GTR	3F

Abbreviations: 3F, triple-F reconstruction (fat, fascia, and flap); IV, third ventricle extension.

approach, the opening of which was extended across the tuberculum sellae to include the planum sphenoidale to provide greater access to the suprasellar space (described previously) (**Fig. 8**).

The first 5 cases were operated before the description of the nasosseptal flap, and the reconstruction to avoid postoperative CSF leak was done with free mucosal graft. Two of these cases (40%) presented postoperative leak that were solved with reoperation.

All the other 13 patients underwent a triple-F reconstruction. Only 1 patient (7.7%) experienced a postoperative CSF leak, which was managed with re-exploration and the flap replaced with success.

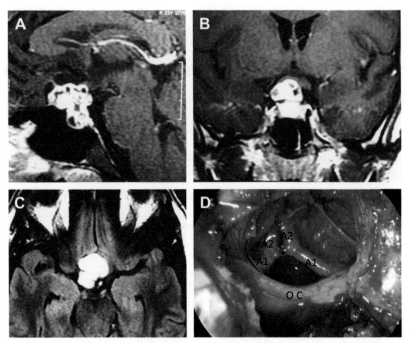

Fig. 7. Case 13. Sagittal (*A*), coronal (*B*), and axial (*C*) T1-weighted MRI with gadolinium of supradiaphragmatic tumor with prechiasmatic position. (*D*) Intraoperative view of the optic chiasm (OC) posteriorly displaced after tumor removal (same case as in *A*, *B*, and *C*). Segments of anterior cerebral artery (A1 and A2) and anterior communicant artery (*asterisk*).

Tumor removal and surgical outcome

GTR (**Figs. 9** and **10**) was achieved in 12 patients (66.7%); 3 of 18 (16.7%) had less than 5% residual tumor, with near total resection (see **Table 4**). Two patients (11.1%) had STR (>70% of removal) and 1 patient had a partial resection (case 9). The rate of patients with satisfatory ressection (ie, GTR + NTR) was 83.4% (15 of 18).

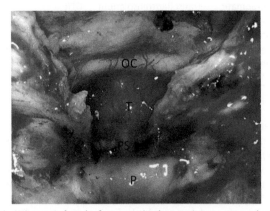

Fig. 8. Case 14. Skull base defect before craniopharyngioma removal. Observe the dural opening, including the planum sphenoidale and the postchiasmatic position of the tumor (T). OC, optic chiasm; PS, pituitary stalk; P, pituitary.

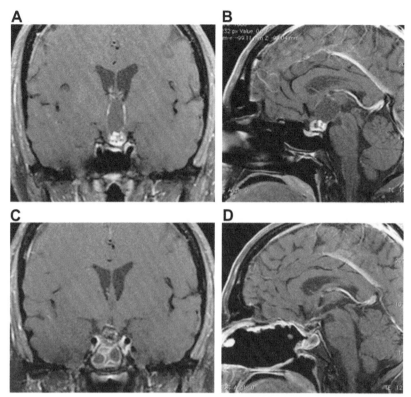

Fig. 9. Case 14. Postchiasmatic, intraventricular tumor. Contrast-enhanced T1-weighted MRI. Preoperative coronal (*A*) and sagittal (*B*) MRI showing a complex craniopharyngioma with suprasellar extension. Postoperative coronal (*C*) and sagittal (*D*) images showing gross total resection.

Postoperative complications

Eight patients (44.4%) had complications. As discussed previously, the authors had 3 cases of CSF leak (16.7%), but in cases in which the flap was used, this rate was 7.7%. One patient (case 6) presented with a hypothalamic syndrome. One patient experienced a residual tumor bleeding (case 9) 3 days after the surgery. The authors re-operated the patient through an external approach. One patient died as a result of a severe hydroelectrolytic disturbance that probably led to a central pontine myelinolysis. One patient experienced meningitis within 48 hours after the surgery, which was confirmed by lumbar puncture and required antibiotics. Finally, the authors had 1 patient who experienced a bilateral visual loss, in addition to hyperphagia and excessive weight gain, in investigation for a presumably hypothalamic dysfunction.

Is Morbidity Decreased in Patients with Endoscopic Resection of Craniopharyngiomas (Vision and Pituitary Function) Compared with Microscopic/Transcranial Surgery?

Any comparison of different case series is of questionable value, because tumors are heterogeneous in anatomic site, consistency, and frequency of infradiaphragmatic location, with distinct postsurgical outcomes.

The mortality rate is much lower in patients undergoing transsphenoidal surgery than in those undergoing transcranial surgery. In recent large transsphenoidal series,

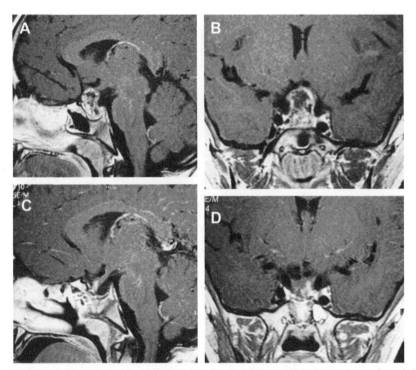

Fig. 10. Case 1. (*A, B*) Preoperative sagittal and coronal T1-weighted MRI views of a subdia-phag- matic craniopharyngioma. (*C, D*) Postoperative sagittal and coronal.

the mortality rate was 0%.[20–24] For transcranial surgery, the rate of early mortality is up to 9%[16,25–27] (EBM grade: C).

In transcranial surgery, the most important source of morbidity is direct damage to the hypothalamus or injury to small perforating arteries.[17]

Comparison of the transcranial and transsphenoidal subgroups in some series showed similar GTR rates[22,27–32] (EBM grade: C).

Given the high risk of recurrence and the high standard of contemporary replacement therapy, radicality should have priority over preservation of endocrine function, especially in young adults and children.[17] Jung and colleagues[28] demonstrated that the preservation of the pituitary stalk provided normal endocrine function in only one-third of patients.

Regarding endocrinologic outcomes, series with endoscopic or classical superior approaches were similar[22,27–32] (EBM grade: C).

Concerning the results of visual function, however, the literature demonstrates a better prognosis after endoscopic transnasal surgery. In Yasargil and colleagues'[27] series of 144 patients, visual improvement was observed in 40.2% of those with preoperative visual field deficits. Similar results were found in superior approaches series: visual deficits improved in 50% and worsened in 33% of patients reported by Jung and colleagues.[28] At 10-year follow-up, 48% of patients from Karavitaki and colleagues' series[30] still had major visual field deficits.

Visual field improvement in endoscopic series was 78% in Jane Jr's and colleagues',[31] 67% in Stamm and colleagues',[22] 78.6% in Campbell and colleagues',[32] and 93% in Gardner and colleagues'[24] (EBM grade: C).

When GTR cannot be safely performed during initial surgery, postoperative external radiation is generally recommended.[11]

EBM Question	Author's reply
Is morbidity decreased in patients with endoscopic resection of craniopharyngiomas (vision, pituitary function) compared to microscopic/trans-cranial surgery?	Visual outcomes are superior in the endoscopic groups. Endocrine outcomes are similar. Mortality rates are higher in trans-cranial surgery compared to a microscopic or endoscopic transphenoidal approach.

REFERENCES

1. Bobustuc GC, Groves MD, Fuller GN. Craniopharyngioma. Neuro-Oncology Perspective 2006. Available at: http://emedicine.medscape.com/article/1157758-overview. Accessed June 9, 2011.
2. Bunin GR, Surawicz TS, Witman PA. The descriptive epidemiology of craniopharyngioma. J Neurosurg 1998;89(4):547–51.
3. Fahlbusch R, Honegger J, Paulus W, et al. Surgical treatment of craniopharyngiomas: experience with 168 patients. J Neurosurg 1999;90:237–50.
4. Parisi J, Mena H. Nonglial tumours. In: Nelson J, Parisi J, Schochet S, editors. Principles and practice of neuropathology. St Louis: Mosby; 1993. p. 203–66.
5. Weiner HL, Wisoff JH, Rosenberg ME, et al. Craniopharyngiomas: a clinicopathological analysis of factors predictive of recurrence and functional outcome. Neurosurgery 1994;35:1001–10.
6. Adamson TE, Wiestler OD, Kleihues P, et al. Correlation of clinical and pathological features in surgically treated craniopharyngiomas. J Neurosurg 1990;73:12–7.
7. Karavitaki N, Cudlip S, Adams CB. Craniopharyngiomas. Endocr Rev 2006;27: 371–97.
8. Hoffman HJ, De Silva M, Humphreys RP, et al. Aggressive surgical management of craniopharyngiomas in children. J Neurosurg 1992;76:47–52.
9. Baskin DS, Wilson CB. Surgical management of craniopharyngiomas. J Neurosurg 1986;65:22–7.
10. Karavitaki N, Wass J. Craniopharyngiomas. Endocrinol Metab Clin North Am 2008;37:173–93.
11. Lund VJ, Stammberger H, Nicolai P, et al. European position paper on endoscopic management of tumours of the nose, paranasal sinuses and skull base. Rhinol Suppl 2010;(22):1–143.
12. Matson D, Crigler J. Management of craniopharyngioma in childhood. J Neurosurg 1969;30:377–90.
13. Laws ER Jr. Transsphenidal microsurgery in the management of craniopharyngioma. J Neurosurg 1980;52:661–6.
14. Wang K, Hong SH, Kim SK, et al. Origin of craniopharyngiomas: implication on the growth pattern. Childs Nerv Syst 2005;21(8–9):628–34.
15. Katz E. Late results of radical excision of craniopharyngiomas in children. J Neurosurg 1975;42:86–90.
16. Di Rocco C, Caldarelli M, Tamburrini G, et al. Surgical management of craniopharyngiomas - experience with a pediatric series. J Pediatr Endocrinol Metab 2006;19:355–66.
17. Honegger J, Tatagiba M. Craniopharyngioma surgery. Pituitary 2008;11(4):361–73.
18. Cavallo LM, Prevedello DM, Solari D, et al. Extended endoscopic endonasal transsphenoidal approach for residual or recurrent craniopharyngiomas. J Neurosurg 2009;111(3):578–89.

19. Stamm AC, Pignatari S, Vellutini E, et al. A novel approach allowing binostril work to the sphenoid sinus. Otolaryngology - Head & Neck Surgery 2008;138(4): 531–2.

20. Maira G, Anile C, Rossi GF, et al. Surgical treatment of craniopharyngiomas: an evaluation of the transsphenoidal and pteronal approaches. Neurosurgery 1995;36:715–24.

21. Chakrabarti I, Amar AP, Couldwell W, et al. Long-term neurological, visual, and endocrine outcomes following transnasal resection of craniopharyngioma. J Neurosurg 2005;102(4):650–7.

22. Stamm AC, Vellutini E, Harvey RJ, et al. Endoscopic transnasal craniotomy and the resection of craniopharyngioma. Laryngoscope 2008;118:1142–8.

23. Jane JA Jr, Prevedello DM, Alden TD, et al. The transsphenoidal resection of pediatric craniopharyngiomas: a case series. J Neurosurg Pediatr 2010;5(1): 49–60.

24. Gardner PA, Kassam AB, Snyderman CH, et al. Outcomes following endoscopic, expanded endonasal resection of suprasellar craniopharyngiomas: a case series. J Neurosurg 2008;108:1043–7.

25. Shi X, Wu B, Zhou ZQ, et al. Microsurgical treatment of craniopharyngiomas: report of 284 patients. Chin Med J (Engl) 2006;119:1653–63.

26. Symon L, Pell MF, Habib AH. Radical excision of craniopharyngioma by the temporal route: a review of 50 patients. Br J Neurosurg 1991;5(6):539–49.

27. Yasargil MG, Curcic M, Kis M, et al. Total removal of craniopharyngiomas. Approaches and long-terms results in 144 patients. J Neurosurg 1990;73:3–11.

28. Jung TY, Jung S, Choi JE, et al. Adult craniopharyngiomas: surgical results with a special focus on endocrinological outcomes and recurrence according to pituitary stalk preservation. J Neurosurg 2009;111(3):572–7.

29. Van-Effenterre R, Boch AL. Craniopharyngioma in adults and children: a study of 122 surgical cases. J Neurosurg 2002;97:3–11.

30. Karavitaki N, Brufani C, Warner JT, et al. Craniopharyngiomas in children and adults: systematic analysis of 121 cases with long-term follow-up. Clin Endocrinol (Oxf) 2005;62(4):397–409.

31. Jane JA Jr, Kiehna E, Payne SC, et al. Early outcomes of endoscopic transsphenoidal surgery for adult craniopharyngiomas. Neurosurg Focus 2010;28(4):1–9.

32. Campbell PG, McGettigan B, Luginbuhl A, et al. Endrocrinological and ophthalmological consequences of an initial endonasal endoscopic approach for resection of craniopharyngiomas. Neurosurg Focus 2010;28(4):E8.

Tuberculum Sella Meningioma

Caroline Hayhurst, MBChB, FRCS, Charles Teo, MBBS, FRACS, AM*

KEYWORDS

- Tuberculum meningioma • Minimally invasive • Endoscopy
- Supraorbital craniotomy • Outcome

Key Points: TUBERCULUM SELLA MENINGIOMA

- Supraorbital craniotomy and expanded endonasal transsphenoidal approach both provide a minimally invasive solution to tuberculum meningiomas.
- Deciding on an approach must take into account specific imaging features in each case.
- Recommendations are based on class C evidence only.

EBM Question	Level of Evidence	Grade of Recommendation
Are visual outcomes better with expanded endonasal transsphenoidal approach than open approaches?	4	C

ANATOMY AND PATHOPHYSIOLOGY

Tuberculum sellae (TS) meningiomas arise from the dura of the TS, chiasmatic sulcus, limbus sphenoidale, and diaphragma sellae. As the TS meningiomas grow in the sub-chiasmal area compressing the optic nerves, they produce quite distinctive clinical, imaging, and microsurgical features. TS meningiomas are often grouped with other

Dr Teo is a consultant for Aesculap, Tuttlingen, Germany.
The Centre for Minimally Invasive Neurosurgery, Suite 3, Level 7, Prince of Wales Private Hospital, Randwick, NSW 2031, Australia
* Corresponding author.
E-mail address: Charlie@neuroendoscopy.info

Otolaryngol Clin N Am 44 (2011) 953–963
doi:10.1016/j.otc.2011.06.012
0030-6665/11/$ – see front matter Crown Copyright © 2011 Published by Elsevier Inc. All rights reserved.

suprasellar and anterior cranial fossa meningiomas, but, because of the distinct dural attachment, TS meningiomas elevate the optic nerves and chiasm, and early optic canal involvement is common. Optic canal involvement is reported in 10% to 90% of TS meningiomas[1–4] and is often appreciated on preoperative imaging in only a small number of patients.

When the tumor is small, the area of dural attachment remains on the TS anterior to the pituitary fossa but may extend to the planum sphenoidale or posteriorly to the diaphragma and infundibulum, with tumor filling the pituitary fossa. In the early stages of growth, the arachnoidal plane is well preserved and the tumor compresses the chiasmatic cistern; however, with further growth, vascular and optic nerve encasement can occur.

CLINICAL PRESENTATION

TS meningiomas commonly present with visual deterioration, even at a small tumor size. The chiasmal syndrome was described by Cushing and Eisenhardt[5] in 1929. This syndrome, as originally described, includes a primary optic atrophy with asymmetric bitemporal field defects in adult patients showing a normal sella on plain skull radiograph and has been the classic characteristic presentation of TS meningiomas. Although the most common pattern of visual disturbance is gradual vision loss in one eye, followed by gradual visual disturbance in the contralateral eye, visual symptoms may sometimes be acute or fluctuating. Other symptoms include headache, anosmia, seizures, and, rarely, pituitary dysfunction.

MANAGEMENT

The primary goal of surgery is maximal tumor resection to improve or at least stabilize visual function. Traditional surgical approaches, such as pterional, subfrontal, and interhemispheric, are familiar to most neurosurgeons, but, in the past decade, minimally invasive techniques have evolved. Both the endonasal endoscopic transsphenoidal approach and the eyebrow keyhole craniotomy have been advocated for TS meningioma,[6–9] both potentially achieving the goals of a minimally invasive technique: minimal access but maximal resection with minimal collateral soft tissue destruction. The definitive choice of a high or low approach for TS meningiomas has been widely debated.[1,10,11] In all patients, the approach should be tailored to the individual case and the specific imaging characteristics, particularly the presence of neurovascular encasement and the lateral extent of the tumor.

EXPANDED ENDONASAL TRANSSPHENOIDAL APPROACH

The expanded endonasal transsphenoidal approach (EETA) has been described extensively.[7,12–15] In brief, the authors perform the procedure entirely under endoscopic vision. The head is placed in Mayfield pin fixation, and image guidance is used throughout (BrainLAB, Westchester, IL, USA). The nasal cavity is packed with lintin strips soaked in 1:2000 adrenaline before draping the field, and, subsequently, the middle turbinate and septal mucosa are infiltrated with 1% bupivacaine with 1:100,000 adrenaline; under endoscopic vision, the middle and superior turbinates are resected. A nasoseptal flap pedicled on the posterior septal branch of the sphenopalatine artery (Hadad-Bassagasteguy flap) is harvested and stored in the nasopharynx for the duration of the procedure. A wide sphenoidotomy is performed after a posterior septectomy. The sella face is then removed, and the bony opening continued through the TS to the planum sphenoidale. The position of the carotids is localized by direct visualization; by frameless stereotaxy; or, when there is bony dehiscence, using a micro-Doppler probe. After bony opening, the dura above and below the diaphragma is coagulated and opened, with control of bleeding from the superior circular sinus with Gelfoam (Pfizer Inc, New York, NY, USA), Floseal (Baxter International Inc, Deerfield, IL, USA), and a bipolar cautery. Further dural coagulation reduces the tumor blood supply and allows internal debulking with minimal obscuration of vision. After tumor volume reduction, the tumor capsule is dissected sharply away from arachnoid attachments and delivered. Both 0° and 30° endoscopes are used during the procedure. After tumor removal, the anterior fossa floor is reconstructed with Duragen (Integra Life Sciences, Boston, MA, USA) and the nasoseptal flap rotated into position. Mucosal to bone flap adherence is maintained with Tisseel (Baxter International Inc, Deerfield, IL, USA) and Gelfoam packing to fill the sphenoid sinus. The Gelfoam is supported with a 14 F Foley catheter left in situ for 48 hours postoperatively. No lumbar drains are used.

TS meningiomas particularly suited to an EETA approach are those that are truly midline with little eccentric lateral growth, those in patients with a large sphenoid sinus, and tumors situated entirely inferior and medial to the optic nerves. Encasement of the optic nerves, carotids, or anterior cerebral artery complex should be sought and excluded on preoperative imaging. In particular, the presence of a cortical cuff separating the tumor capsule from the anterior cerebral arteries is an excellent marker that vascular encasement is unlikely to be encountered (**Fig. 1**). The advantages and disadvantages of the EETA are listed in **Box 1**.

EYEBROW SUPRAORBITAL KEYHOLE CRANIOTOMY

This technique has been well described.[6,10] In brief, following the induction of general anesthesia, the head is placed in the Mayfield pin fixation with the head turned 30° to the contralateral side and the head extended to bring the malar uppermost. The side of the approach is determined by the lateral projection of the tumor. The skin incision is placed in the upper border of the eyebrow, medial to the supraorbital nerve (**Fig. 2**A). After skin and muscle dissections, which are retracted superiorly using fishhooks, a pericranial flap is reflected inferiorly and the keyhole exposed. A single burr hole is made at the keyhole, and a free supraorbital bone flap is made approximately 20 mm in height (or the equivalent of the width of an open bipolar shaft). The inner table of the supraorbital rim is then drilled down along with the bony protuberances of the anterior fossa floor to gain additional exposure (see **Fig. 2**B). The dura is opened in

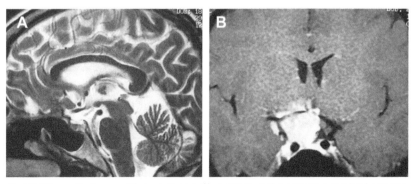

Fig. 1. (*A*) TS meningioma with a cortical cuff separating the anterior cerebral arteries. (*B*) Midline TS meningioma with vascular encasement.

Box 1
Advantages and disadvantages of the EETA approach

Advantages

    No incisions

    Faster recovery

    Early devascularization of tumor

    No brain retraction

    Minimal manipulation of optic apparatus

Disadvantages

    Risk of cerebrospinal fluid leak

    Potential loss of olfaction

    Difficult to remove tumor in optic canal when superolateral to optic nerve

    Difficult to dissect adherent/encased small vessels at posterior margin

---

a C-shaped manner and reflected inferiorly. Under microscopic vision, the arachnoid of the carotid cistern is identified and opened to allow cerebrospinal fluid (CSF) release. No fixed brain retraction is used. Standard microsurgical techniques of tumor removal are used and the optic canals opened when required for complete tumor removal and decompression of the optic nerves. After tumor removal, the dura is closed watertight and the bone flap replaced using 2 Craniofix clamps (Aesculap Inc, Center Valley, PA, USA). The bone flap is approximated flush to the upper border of the craniotomy and the resulting inferior margin bone defect filled with Surgicel (Ethicon Inc, Johnson and Johnson, Piscataway, NJ, USA), to reduce depressions in the forehead. The pericranial flap is carefully reapproximated, and the galea and skin are closed without tension. A subcuticular nylon running suture provides the best cosmetic outcome for skin closure.

TS meningiomas for which an eyebrow approach would be most suitable are those with the tumor extending lateral to the carotid artery or superior and lateral to the optic nerves. Patients with normal pituitary function may also be considered preferentially for the eyebrow approach. In addition, better microsurgical control of adherent or encased vessels can be achieved. The advantages and disadvantages of the eyebrow approach are listed in **Box 2**.

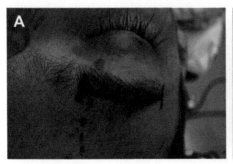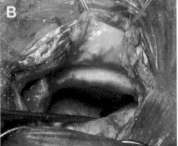

Fig. 2. Eyebrow approach. (*A*) Skin incision. (*B*) Extent of exposure after craniotomy.

Box 2
Advantages and disadvantages of the eyebrow approach

Advantages

    Rapid access

    Low risk of CSF leak

    Good access to optic canals

    Standard microsurgical dissection technique

Disadvantages

    Breach of frontal sinus if large

    Brain retraction

    Difficult to remove tumor if it extends anterior to planum

---

In some cases, a combined endonasal and supraorbital approach may be warranted, particularly in situations in which there is tumor extending anterior to the planum and tumor filling the sella and a trajectory from both above and below is required for complete tumor resection (**Figs. 3** and **4**).

LITERATURE REVIEW
Are Visual Outcomes Better with EETA than Open Approaches

Any new technique must demonstrate at least equal outcomes to existing surgical approaches. Reports of extent of tumor resection with standard microsurgical approaches range from 66% to 100%,[16–21] with visual outcome reported as improved or stable in 25% to 80%.[17,19,21] Visual outcome is partially dependent on tumor size, with a worse reported outcome in tumors larger than 3 cm.[22] In addition, the duration of visual deterioration influences outcome, with those patients with visual symptoms for less than 12 months demonstrating better visual outcome,[23,24] making a direct comparison of results difficult.

Conversely, postoperative visual deterioration has been reported in up to 20% of patients in standard microsurgical series.[17,25] The mechanism of visual deterioration postoperatively is either a direct effect of optic nerve manipulation or devascularization of the nerve.[26]

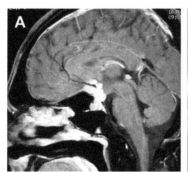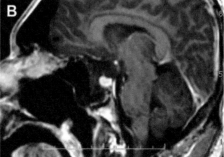

Fig. 3. Combined approach. (*A*) TS meningioma with anterior and posterior extension; note the vascular encasement. (*B*) Complete tumor resection after a combined EETA and supraorbital craniotomy.

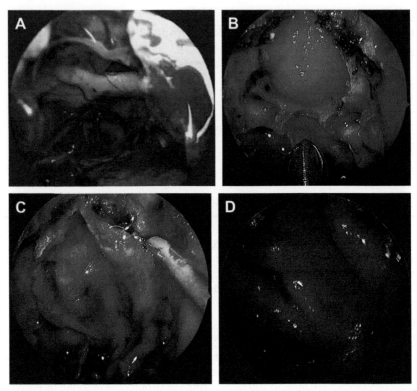

Fig. 4. Endoscopic TS meningioma removal. (*A*) Indentation of inferomedial optic nerve after tumor removal from below. (*B*) Completed nasoseptal flap repair with Duragen (Integra Life Sciences, Boston, MA, USA) underlay. (*C*) Flap before fibrin glue application. (*D*) Three weeks postoperatively.

The body of evidence on outcomes following minimally invasive approaches for suprasellar meningiomas remains sparse and is based on retrospective case series. When considering a purely endoscopic endonasal transsphenoidal approach to specifically TS meningiomas, a total of 38 cases have been reported.[7,11,13–15,27–29] The patient characteristics and outcomes for all reported EETAs for TS meningiomas in the English literature are summarized in **Table 1**. In addition, Fatemi and colleagues[10] and Kitano and colleagues[8] report case series of endonasal removal of TS meningiomas using a microscope. Similarly, there are few reports of outcome following supraorbital keyhole craniotomy for TS meningioma.[1,6,30–32] Kitano and colleagues[8] and de Divitiis and colleagues[11] compare consecutive cohorts of TS meningioma operated via standard pterional or frontal craniotomies and transsphenoidal approaches. Fatemi and colleagues[10] report on a retrospective consecutive cohort of patients with TS meningioma, directly comparing the transsphenoidal approach with the supraorbital keyhole approach.

Extent of Resection

Of the 38 combined reported cases of a purely endoscopic transsphenoidal approach, the overall complete resection rate is 84% (see **Table 1**).[7,13–15,27,28] The site of residual disease is most often the optic canal or adherent to the anterior cerebral artery

Table 1
Reported case series of purely endoscopic EETA for TS meningioma

Authors	Year of Publication	Number of Patients	Tumor Size	Presenting Symptoms	Gross Total Resection	Site of Residual Disease	Vascular Encasement	CSF Leak Rate	Reconstruction Technique	Visual Outcome	Endocrine
Wang et al[28]	2010	12	2–4 cm	Visual deterioration, 11; headaches, 1	11 (92%)	Optic canal	1	1/12 (8%)	Fat and dural substitute	Improved, 11; unchanged, 1	Transient DI, 1/12 (8%)
Ceylan et al[27]	2009	2	2–4 cm	—	1 (50%)	Cisternal	No	5/13 (38%)	Mixed	—	Transient DI, 3/13 (23%)
de Devitiis et al[29]	2008	7	1.4–3.8 cm	Visual deterioration, 7	6 (86%)	Optic canal	No[b]	2/7 (29%)	Mixed	Improved, 5; unchanged, 2; transient worsening, 3	Transient DI, 1/7 (14%)
Dehdashti et al[14]	2009	1	2.6 cm	Visual deterioration	1 (100%)	—	No	1 (100%)	Fascia lata + fat	Improved	None
Gardner et al[7]	2008	13	1.4–38.3 mL[a]	Visual deterioration, 10; headaches, 1; incidental, 1; prior residual tumor, 1	11/13 (85%)	—	—	8/13 (62%)	Mixed	Improved 100%	None
Laufer et al[15]	2007	3	2–3.5 cm	Visual deterioration	2 (66%)	ACoA	1	1/3 (33%)	Fascia lata + glue	Improved 100%	Permanent DI, 1/3 (33%)

Abbreviations: ACoA, anterior communicating artery; DI, diabetes insipidus.
[a] Reported volume.
[b] One death in the series because of intraventricular hemorrhage.

complex.[15,28,33] Fatemi and colleagues[10] report complete tumor resection in 50% of the cases using a microscopic endoscope-assisted approach, but residual disease was only seen in those with prior surgery, prior radiotherapy, or vascular encasement. Other case series using a microscopic endonasal approach report complete resection in 57% to 100%.[9,34–36]

Using a supraorbital craniotomy in 58 patients with TS meningioma, Mahmoud and colleagues[1] achieved a complete resection in 87.9%. The site of residual disease is not stated in this series. Smaller case series using a supraorbital keyhole craniotomy report complete resection in 22% to 100% of patients.[6,10,31,32]

Visual Outcome

Several case series define postoperative visual status as improved, unchanged, or worse. Using these parameters, improvement or stability of vision is reported in 100% of the cases in the purely endoscopic transsphenoidal series in which visual outcome is reported.[7,13–15,28] de Divitiis and colleagues[13] report transient worsening in 3 patients after endoscopic endonasal removal of TS meningioma. Fatemi and colleagues[10] report improvement of vision in 10 of 11 patients with preoperative visual deterioration and worsening of vision in 1 patient after microscopic transsphenoidal resection.

Kitano and colleagues[8] report an in-depth analysis of visual acuity and visual field defects after either a standard transcranial approach or a microscopic transsphenoidal approach in 28 patients with TS meningioma. The investigators found a significant difference in the rate of improvement of visual acuity between the transsphenoidal and transcranial group, with improvement in acuity in 59% and 25%, respectively. There was no difference in the rate of improvement of visual field defects between the approaches, 38% in both groups. In addition, there was no significant difference in the rate of visual worsening in either the transcranial or the transsphenoidal group.

Similarly, Mahmoud and colleagues[1] report a comprehensive assessment of visual outcome after supraorbital craniotomy for TS meningioma. Of the 39 patients in whom the German Ophthalmologic Society (GOS) scale was used to grade both visual acuity and visual fields, 29 (74%) showed improvement in the visual impairment score postoperatively and 7 (18%) showed no change. Visual acuity was normalized in 20%. In this series, 3 patients (8%) had deterioration in vision after surgery.

Wang and colleagues[28] also report visual outcome based on the GOS visual impairment score for 12 patients who underwent purely endoscopic EETA. In their series, 5 patients (41%) had normalization of visual acuity and visual fields postoperatively. Eleven patients improved, and 1 was unchanged. No patients experienced visual deterioration after surgery.

Series of TS meningioma resection with a standard craniotomy show visual deterioration in approximately 20% of cases.[17,21,25,37,38] On this basis, it would seem that visual outcomes are superior using an endonasal transsphenoidal approach, in terms of visual improvement and avoiding visual deterioration. This outcome suggests that the degree of optic nerve manipulation and avoidance of the perforating artery supply to the superior surface of the optic apparatus are crucial to visual preservation.

Complications

The endonasal transsphenoidal approach is accompanied by a need for an extensive skull base reconstruction to avoid CSF leak and the potential need for reintervention. The case series of EETA for TS meningioma resection have included a variety of reconstruction methods, including abdominal fat and dural substitute,[28] titanium mesh buttress and fat,[10] and the pedicled nasoseptal flap.[7] The CSF leak rate is extremely variable (see **Table 1**). Gardner and colleagues[7] report a CSF leak rate of 62% for TS meningioma. However, after the introduction of the nasoseptal flap, the CSF leak rate for expanded endonasal procedures has decreased from 40% to 5.4%.[7,39] Harvey and colleagues[39] report a CSF leak rate of 3.3% after the closure of large skull base defects with a posterior septal pedicled flap. In the supraorbital craniotomy series by Fatemi and colleagues,[10] the CSF leak rate is 7%.

No series on TS meningioma resection report any anterior pituitary dysfunction, but posterior pituitary dysfunction is reported in 7% to 33% of EETA cases.[10,15,27,28,33] Mahmoud and colleagues[1] report 2 cases (3%) of transient diabetes insipidus after a supraorbital craniotomy for TS meningioma.

Postoperative anosmia has not been reported in the purely endoscopic EETA series, but Mahmoud and colleagues[1] report anosmia in 5% of cases after supraorbital craniotomy, and Kitano and colleagues[8] noted anosmia in 12.5% of patients after microscopic EETA. Also Kitano and colleagues[8] reported perforating artery infarction in 3 transcranial cases (25%) and 2 transsphenoidal cases (12.5%), although without focal neurologic deficit.

SUMMARY

Any surgical approach should be tailored to the individual case, and the best approach is the one that achieves complete curative tumor resection with the least operative morbidity. In the case of TS meningioma, this approach depends on the relationship of the tumor with the optic nerves, optic canal, and anterior cerebral artery complex. Evidence based on retrospective small case series suggests that visual outcomes are superior using an endonasal transsphenoidal approach (grade C, retrospective cohorts and case series). The extent of resection achieved is comparable using a transcranial or endonasal approach.

EBM Question	Author's reply
Are visual outcomes better with expanded endonasal transsphenoidal approach than open approaches?	Limited evidence suggests visual outcomes are better in both expanded endonasal transsphenoidal and supra-orbital approaches compared to traditional trans-cranial surgery

REFERENCES

1. Mahmoud M, Nader R, Al-Mefty O. Optic canal involvement in tuberculum sellae meningiomas: influence on approach, recurrence, and visual recovery. Neurosurgery 2010;67(Suppl Operative 3):108–18 [discussion: 118–109].
2. Margalit NS, Lesser JB, Moche J, et al. Meningiomas involving the optic nerve: technical aspects and outcomes for a series of 50 patients. Neurosurgery 2003;53(3):523–32 [discussion: 532–523].
3. Arai H, Sato K, Okuda, et al. Transcranial transsphenoidal approach for tuberculum sellae meningiomas. Acta Neurochir (Wien) 2000;142(7):751–6 [discussion: 756–7].
4. Sade B, Lee JH. High incidence of optic canal involvement in tuberculum sellae meningiomas: rationale for aggressive skull base approach. Surg Neurol 2009; 72(2):118–23 [discussion: 123].

5. Cushing H, Eisenhardt L. Meningiomas arising from the tuberculum sellae, with syndrome of primary optic atropy bitemporal field defects combined with normal sellae turcica in a middle aged person. Arch Opthalmol 1929;1(41):168–206.

6. Fernandes YB, Maitrot D, Kehrli P, et al. Supraorbital eyebrow approach to skull base lesions. Arq Neuropsiquiatr 2002;60(2-A):246–50.

7. Gardner PA, Kassam AB, Thomas A, et al. Endoscopic endonasal resection of anterior cranial base meningiomas. Neurosurgery 2008;63(1):36–52 [discussion: 52–34].

8. Kitano M, Taneda M, Nakao Y. Postoperative improvement in visual function in patients with tuberculum sellae meningiomas: results of the extended transsphenoidal and transcranial approaches. J Neurosurg 2007;107(2):337–46.

9. Couldwell WT, Weiss MH, Rabb C, et al. Variations on the standard transsphenoidal approach to the sellar region, with emphasis on the extended approaches and parasellar approaches: surgical experience in 105 cases. Neurosurgery 2004;55(3):539–47 [discussion: 547–50].

10. Fatemi N, Dusick JR, de Paiva Neto MA, et al. Endonasal versus supraorbital keyhole removal of craniopharyngiomas and tuberculum sellae meningiomas. Neurosurgery 2009;64(5 Suppl 2):269–84 [discussion: 284–6].

11. de Divitiis E, Esposito F, Cappabianca P, et al. Tuberculum sellae meningiomas: high route or low route? A series of 51 consecutive cases. Neurosurgery 2008; 62(3):556–63 [discussion: 556–63].

12. de Divitiis E, Cavallo LM, Cappabianca P, et al. Extended endoscopic endonasal transsphenoidal approach for the removal of suprasellar tumors: part 2. Neurosurgery 2007;60(1):46–58 [discussion: 58–49].

13. de Divitiis E, Cavallo LM, Esposito F, et al. Extended endoscopic transsphenoidal approach for tuberculum sellae meningiomas. Neurosurgery 2007;61(5 Suppl 2): 229–37 [discussion: 237–228].

14. Dehdashti AR, Ganna A, Witterick I, et al. Expanded endoscopic endonasal approach for anterior cranial base and suprasellar lesions: indications and limitations. Neurosurgery 2009;64(4):677–87 [discussion: 687–679].

15. Laufer I, Anand VK, Schwartz TH. Endoscopic, endonasal extended transsphenoidal, transplanum transtuberculum approach for resection of suprasellar lesions. J Neurosurg 2007;106(3):400–6.

16. Al-Mefty O, Holoubi A, Rifai A, et al. Microsurgical removal of suprasellar meningiomas. Neurosurgery 1985;16(3):364–72.

17. Fahlbusch R, Schott W. Pterional surgery of meningiomas of the tuberculum sellae and planum sphenoidale: surgical results with special consideration of ophthalmological and endocrinological outcomes. J Neurosurg 2002;96(2):235–43.

18. Kinjo T, al-Mefty O, Ciric I. Diaphragma sellae meningiomas. Neurosurgery 1995; 36(6):1082–92.

19. Goel A, Muzumdar D, Desai KI. Tuberculum sellae meningioma: a report on management on the basis of a surgical experience with 70 patients. Neurosurgery 2002;51(6):1358–63 [discussion: 1363–1354].

20. Grisoli F, Diaz-Vasquez P, Riss M, et al. Microsurgical management of tuberculum sellae meningiomas. Results in 28 consecutive cases. Surg Neurol 1986;26(1): 37–44.

21. Jallo GI, Benjamin V. Tuberculum sellae meningiomas: microsurgical anatomy and surgical technique. Neurosurgery 2002;51(6):1432–9 [discussion: 1439–40].

22. Li-Hua C, Ling C, Li-Xu L. Microsurgical management of tuberculum sellae meningiomas by the frontolateral approach: surgical technique and visual outcome. Clin Neurol Neurosurg 2011;113(1):39–47.

23. Kim TW, Jung S, Jung TY, et al. Prognostic factors of postoperative visual outcomes in tuberculum sellae meningioma. Br J Neurosurg 2008;22(2):231–4.
24. Rosenstein J, Symon L. Surgical management of suprasellar meningioma. Part 2: prognosis for visual function following craniotomy. J Neurosurg 1984;61(4):642–8.
25. Pamir MN, Ozduman K, Belirgen M, et al. Outcome determinants of pterional surgery for tuberculum sellae meningiomas. Acta Neurochir (Wien) 2005;147(11): 1121–30 [discussion: 1130].
26. Li X, Liu M, Liu Y, et al. Surgical management of tuberculum sellae meningiomas. J Clin Neurosci 2007;14(12):1150–4.
27. Ceylan S, Koc K, Anik I. Extended endoscopic approaches for midline skull-base lesions. Neurosurg Rev 2009;32(3):309–19 [discussion: 318–309].
28. Wang Q, Lu XJ, Ji WY, et al. Visual outcome after extended endoscopic endonasal transphenoidal surgery for tuberculum sella meningiomas. World Neurosurg 2010;73(6):694–700.
29. de Divitiis E, Esposito F, Cappabianca P, et al. Endoscopic transnasal resection of anterior cranial fossa meningiomas. Neurosurg Focus 2008;25(6):E8.
30. de Paiva-Neto MA, de Tella OI Jr. Supra-orbital keyhole removal of anterior fossa and parasellar meningiomas. Arq Neuropsiquiatr 2010;68(3):418–23.
31. Zhang MZ, Wang L, Zhang W, et al. The supraorbital keyhole approach with eyebrow incisions for treating lesions in the anterior fossa and sellar region. Chin Med J (Engl) 2004;117(3):323–6.
32. Wiedemayer H, Sandalcioglu IE, Wiedemayer H, et al. The supraorbital keyhole approach via an eyebrow incision for resection of tumors around the sella and the anterior skull base. Minim Invasive Neurosurg 2004;47(4):221–5.
33. de Divitiis E, Cavallo LM, Esposito F, et al. Extended endoscopic transsphenoidal approach for tuberculum sellae meningiomas. Neurosurgery 2008;62(6 Suppl 3): 1192–201.
34. Kaptain GJ, Vincent DA, Sheehan JP, et al. Transsphenoidal approaches for the extracapsular resection of midline suprasellar and anterior cranial base lesions. Neurosurgery 2001;49(1):94–100 [discussion 100–1].
35. Cook SW, Smith Z, Kelly DF. Endonasal transsphenoidal removal of tuberculum sellae meningiomas: technical note. Neurosurgery 2004;55(1):239–44 [discussion 244–36].
36. Dusick JR, Esposito F, Kelly DF, et al. The extended direct endonasal transsphenoidal approach for nonadenomatous suprasellar tumors. J Neurosurg 2005; 102(5):832–41.
37. Bassiouni H, Asgari S, Stolke D. Tuberculum sellae meningiomas: functional outcome in a consecutive series treated microsurgically. Surg Neurol 2006; 66(1):37–44 [discussion 44–35].
38. Park CK, Jung HW, Yang SY, et al. Surgically treated tuberculum sellae and diaphragm sellae meningiomas: the importance of short-term visual outcome. Neurosurgery 2006;59(2):238–43 [discussion 238–43].
39. Harvey RJ, Nogueira JF, Schlosser RJ, et al. Closure of large skull base defects after endoscopic transnasal craniotomy. Clinical article. J Neurosurg 2009; 111(2):371–9.

Olfactory Groove Meningioma

Nithin D. Adappa, MD[a,*], John Y.K. Lee, MD[b],
Alexander G. Chiu, MD[c], James N. Palmer, MD[a]

KEYWORDS

• Endoscopic • Skull Base • Sinus • Tumor • Paranasal

Key Points: OLFACTORY GROOVE MENINGIOMA

• Because of their slow growth, olfactory groove meningiomas (OGMs) often present late as large intracranial lesions.

• Diagnosis requires a thorough history and physical examination including nasal endoscopy in conjunction with radiographic imaging.

• OGMs are treated primarily with surgical resection. There are several surgical approaches for resection. Endoscopic resection continues to garner further interest as a minimally invasive resection technique, although long-term follow-up data are still necessary.

• If unable to perform surgery, or the patient presents with recurrence, other treatment modalities may be applied. These treatments include radiation therapy, stereotactic radiosurgery (SRS), and chemotherapy.

• Currently, several trials are underway evaluating targeted molecular therapy in meningioma treatment.

EBM Question	Level of Evidence	Grade of Recommendation
Is the morbidity of an endoscopic approach less than an open approach for OGM resection?	4	C

Disclosures: Nithin D. Adappa, none. John Y.K. Lee, Consultant Stryker. Alex G. Chiu, Consultant BrainLAB, Olympus Gyrus, and royalties from NeilMED. James N. Palmer, Consultant Gyrus/Olympus, OptiNose, Alcon, and royalties from ForSinuses.
[a] Department of Otorhinolaryngology–Head and Neck Surgery, University of Pennsylvania School of Medicine, Hospital of the University of Pennsylvania, Ravdin Building 5th Floor, 3400 Spruce Street, Philadelphia, PA 19104, USA
[b] Department of Neurosurgery, University of Pennsylvania School of Medicine, Hospital of the University of Pennsylvania, 235 South 8th Street, Philadelphia, PA 19104, USA
[c] Division of Otolaryngology–Head and Neck Surgery, Arizona Health Science Center, University of Arizona, PO Box 245074, 1501 North Campbell Avenue, Tucson, AZ 85724-5074, USA
* Corresponding author.
E-mail address: Nithin.Adappa@uphs.upenn.edu

Otolaryngol Clin N Am 44 (2011) 965–980
doi:10.1016/j.otc.2011.06.001
0030-6665/11/$ – see front matter © 2011 Elsevier Inc. All rights reserved.

Meningiomas are usually slow-growing benign tumors that are believed to develop from the arachnoidal cap cells. Diagnosis is based on an accurate history and physical examination, including nasal endoscopy, because up to 15% of patients are reported to have an intranasal component.[1] They account for approximately 20% of primary intracranial tumors and OGMs account for 10% of intracranial meningiomas.[2]

They were first described in 1835 in Cruveilhier's *Traite d'Anatomie*.[3] An Italian surgeon, Francesco Durante, in 1885 described the first successful resection of an OGM. In 1938, Cushing[4] reported a series of 28 cases resected through a unilateral frontal craniotomy and subfrontal approach. He had a mortality rate of 19%.[3]

OGMs must be differentiated from other anterior cranial fossa meningiomas as well as other intracranial neoplasms. They differ in presentation, neurologic findings, operative approaches, postoperative outcomes, complications, and overall morbidity and morality.

EPIDEMIOLOGY OF MENINGIOMAS

The prevalence of pathologically confirmed meningiomas is estimated to be approximately 97.5 in 100,000 in the United States, with more than 170,000 individuals currently diagnosed. There is a 2:1 female/male ratio. There have been an increasing number of diagnosed patients in the past several decades. It is unclear whether this is a real trend or a bias from increasingly accurate and more easily obtainable imaging studies.[5]

PATHOPHYSIOLOGY OF MENINGIOMAS

Meningiomas are believed to arise from the meningothelial cap cells that are normally distributed through the arachnoid trabeculations.[6] The greatest concentration of meningothelial cells is found in the arachnoid villi at the dural sinuses, cranial nerve foramina, middle cranial fossa, and the cribriform plate. Subsequently, meningiomas are commonly found over the convexity, along the falx, and at the skull base. The tumors are generally encapsulated and attached to dura. The dura provides some blood supply, but OGMs primarily receive their vascular supply from the anterior and posterior ethmoidal arteries. Histologically, they appear benign, presenting with typical features, including whorls of arachnoid cells surrounding a central hyaline material that eventually calcifies to form psammoma bodies. The cells are arranged in sheaths separated by connective tissue trabeculae.[7]

There are several meningioma subtypes, including meningotheliomatous, fibrous, and transitional types (also known as psammomatous tumors). The subtype provides little prognostic value. The only subtypes that have true clinical relevance are clear cell meningiomas, because they behave more aggressively; secretory meningiomas, which secrete vascular endothelial growth factor (VEGF) and are associated with marked edema; and papillary or rhabdoid variants, which are treated as malignant tumors. Norden and colleagues[8] describe the recurrence rate and median survival based on WHO classification system. Meningiomas are classified based on the World Health Organization grading system (**Table 1**).[9] Malignant meningiomas are rare, but half of these patients develop distant metastases, most commonly to bone, liver, or lung (**Fig. 1**).[7]

Meningiomas are typically associated with 1 or more focal chromosomal deletion(s), and atypical and malignant grades tend to have multiple chromosomal copy number alterations consistent with the acquisition of mutations that foster genomic instability.[10,11]

Table 1
Survival and recurrence rates by World Health Organization histologic grade

WHO Grade	Meningiomas (%)	Recurrence Rate (%)[60]	Median Survival (Y)
I (benign)	90	7–20	>10[61,62]
II (atypical)	5–7	40	11.5[63]
III (malignant)	<3	50–80	2.7[63]

Data from Louis DN, Budka H, von Deimling A, et al. In: Kielhues P, Cavanee WK, editors. World Health Organization classification of tumours. Pathology and genetics of tumours of the nervous system. Lyon (France): IARC Press; 2000. p. 176–84.

Deletion and inactivation of NF2 on chromosome 22 is a predominant feature in sporadic meningiomas.[12] Additional genes are likely involved as well, because loss of NF2 occurs in only one-third of patients who exhibit loss of heterozygosity of chromosome 22.[13] Additional genomic regions that are recurrently lost in meningiomas include 14q, 1p, 6q, and 18q.[14] Meningiomas with increased tumor grade are found to have increased genetic alterations.[15] In general, a small number of mutations may be necessary for most meningiomas. The difficulty with meningiomas is the long latency periods of the tumors, which lead to the challenges in identifying the source and timing of the initiating mutations.

RISK FACTORS FOR MENINGIOMA

Currently, the primary environmental risk factor identified for meningiomas is exposure to ionizing radiation. Studies have shown a sixfold to tenfold increase in meningioma formation.[16–19] The best example is atomic bomb survivors who displayed a significantly increased risk for meningioma.[20] Evidence also shows increased risk at lower dose levels. Between 1948 and 1960, children in Israel were treated with ionizing radiation for tinea capitis.[21] They have a relative risk of almost 10 for meningioma development.

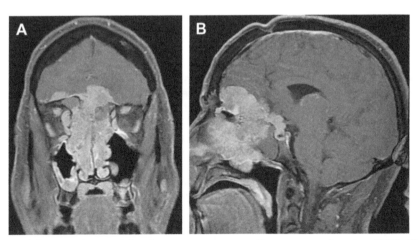

Fig. 1. (*A*) Coronal T1-weighted postcontrast magnetic resonance imaging (MRI). This patient previously had a resection of an OGM. He was disease free for greater than 5 years but, in a period of 6 months, rapidly developed a malignant meningioma and ultimately died without additional treatment. (*B*) Sagittal T1-weighted postcontrast MRI of malignant meningioma from (*A*). (*Images courtesy of* Dr Richard Harvey.)

There is also an association between hormones and the risk for meningioma development. This association was initially suggested because of the observation of increased incidence of postpubertal disease in women versus men. As previously mentioned, there is a 2:1 female/male ratio with a peak ratio of 3.15:1 during peak reproductive years.[22] In addition, some meningiomas present histologically with estrogen, progesterone, and androgen receptors.[22,23] Studies have shown progesterone receptors on 80% of meningiomas in woman and in 40% of those in men.[7] Furthermore, there is an association between breast cancer and meningiomas. In conjunction with studies showing that some meningiomas change size during different phases of the menstrual cycle and pregnancy, and the regression of multiple meningiomas in patients following cessation of estrogen agonist therapy, this has led to numerous investigational trials.[22,23]

Despite the data correlating hormones with meningiomas, they have not been consistently associated with meningioma incidence. The significance of hormone receptors expressed on meningiomas is still a matter of debate and its significance is still unclear. Several future studies are dedicated to evaluating these hormone receptors with a goal of improving treatment, much as hormone receptor treatment has revolutionized breast cancer therapy.

Head trauma has also been suggested by some as a risk factor for meningiomas. Small case-control studies have reported an increased risk of meningioma associated with head trauma to both men and women.[24,25] Conversely, there have been other studies that have found no such association.[26,27]

With several reports identifying a relationship between glial brain tumors and allergic disease such as asthma and eczema, this corollary has been studied with meningiomas. Little evidence has been found to support this. In addition, no occupationally or industrially exposed groups of patients have identified any clear association.[22,28]

There have been some studies of the relationship between meningioma risk and family history. Between 1% and 3% of the adult population may have a meningioma.[29,30] Despite this, families with multiple members diagnosed with meningioma are rare. If families have any association, this is believed to be caused by inherited NF2 mutations. Currently, no family-based genetic linkage has been reported.

ANATOMY

OGMs arise in the midline over the cribriform plate and frontosphenoidal suture. Although they generally arise in the midline, they may extend predominantly to one side. Most of these tumors occupy the floor of the anterior cranial fossa extending from the crista galli to the tuberculum sella.[31] Extension into the ethmoid sinuses have been shown in 15% of cases (**Fig. 2**).[1] Further extension into the nasal cavity and orbit has been reported. Similarities exist between posteriorly extending OGMs and tuberculum sellae meningiomas. The main difference between the 2 is the location of the optic apparatus in relationship to the tumor.[6] OGMs push the optic nerves and the chiasm downward and posteriorly as they grow.[32] Conversely, tuberculum sellae meningiomas elevate the chiasm and displace the optic nerve superolaterally because these neoplasms occupy the subchiasmal position. The blood supply to OGMs is commonly derived from the anterior and posterior ethmoidal arteries. In addition, they receive contributions from the anterior branches of the middle meningeal artery and the meningeal branches of the ophthalmic artery. If the tumor is extensive in size, vascular supply from small branches of the anterior communication artery are common.[33]

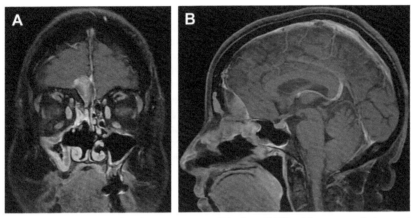

Fig. 2. (*A*) Coronal T1-weighted postcontrast MRI of an OGM with paranasal sinus extension. (*B*) Sagittal T1-weighted postcontrast MRI showing the same OGM with paranasal sinus extension. (*Images courtesy of* Dr Richard Harvey.)

PRESENTATION AND WORK-UP

Because of the slow growth and the location of OGMs, clinical presentation is generally delayed. The most common presenting symptom is olfactory impairment (58.8%), followed by headache, visual impairment, and mental status changes (**Box 1**).[34]

Diagnosis is generally made based on radiographic imaging. Magnetic resonance imaging (MRI) is the imaging modality of choice. Before the widespread use of MRI, angiography was used to suggest the diagnosis based on showing arterial supply from anterior and posterior ethmoidal arteries and the delayed vascular blush that is

Box 1
Presenting signs and symptoms of OGMs
Mental status changes
Olfactory impairment
Headache
Nasal obstruction
Visual impairment
Papilledema
Epilepsy
Motor deficit
Optic nerve atrophy
Incontinence
Foster Kennedy
Sinusitis
Exophthalmos
Telecanthus

characteristic of OGMs. MRI is generally preferred because it can show the dural origin of the tumor in most cases. OGMs are typically isointense or hypointense to gray matter on T1-weighted images and isointense or hyperintense on T2-weighted images. In addition, they have a strong homogeneous enhancement with gadolinium. Most meningiomas show a characteristic marginal dural thickening that tapers peripherally (often termed the dural tail). On computed tomography (CT), OGMs typically appear as a well-defined extra-axial mass that displaces the normal brain. They are smooth in contour, adjacent to dural structures, and often are calcified or multilobulated. Noncontrast CT shows isointensity with normal surrounding brain parenchyma and makes diagnosis difficult. With intravenous contrast, OGMs present with uniform enhancement. Approximately 15% of cases present with an atypical pattern of necrosis, cyst formation, or hemorrhage.[7]

MANAGEMENT OF MENINGIOMAS

Treatment options for OGMs are similar to other skull base tumors. For small tumors in elderly or medically ill patients, observation with serial imaging may be acceptable. Definitive therapy for OGMs is surgical, but other options include radiation therapy (RT), and SRS. Investigational studies in chemotherapy and targeted molecular therapy are ongoing.

OGMs are often large at the time of presentation because of their slow, indolent growth. In some series, 50% to 60% of OGMs were larger than 6 cm in diameter at the time of surgery.[6,35] Despite the large size, complete resection is generally possible. OGMs have an arachnoid membrane separating the tumor from nearly all critical neurovascular structures, which facilitates a complete resection.

SURGICAL THERAPY

Since Cushing described surgical resection of OGMs using a unilateral frontal craniotomy, numerous approaches have been described for definitive therapy. Today, commonly described approaches include wide bifrontal craniotomy with subfrontal approach, unilateral frontal craniotomy with subfrontal approach, pterional approach, and endoscopic approach.

This article outlines the advantages and disadvantages of all the neurosurgical approaches, but focuses on the technical aspects of the endoscopic approach.

The bifrontal craniotomy with subfrontal approach provides wide exposure for radical tumor resection, drilling of hyperostosis in the cribriform plate area of the planum sphenoidale and tuberculum sellae, and unroofing the optic nerves if necessary. The disadvantages to this procedure include significant brain retraction. With large tumors, brain edema can result in the brain herniating into the craniotomy window, often requiring partial resection of the frontal lobe. In addition, critical anatomic structures, including the optic apparatus, carotids, and the anterior communicating complex, present late in the dissection.

The unilateral frontal craniotomy with subfrontal approach has the advantage compared with the previously mentioned procedure that it spares the contralateral frontal lobe and superior sagittal sinus. The disadvantages are similar to the bifrontal craniotomy. In addition, this approach provides a smaller opening with a narrow view via a unilateral approach.

The pterional approach is considered a new approach to OGMs.[35,36] This approach provides several advantages compared with other open approaches. It is less invasive than a bifrontal craniotomy. In addition, it avoids cerebrospinal fluid (CSF) leaks, because the frontal sinus is not transected. The optic nerve can also be localized and secured before tumor manipulation. The ipsilateral internal carotid artery also comes into view early in the dissection. The major disadvantage to this approach is that it uses a narrow working angle. In patients with a high-riding tumor, the upper portion is in a relatively blind area, and may require significant brain retraction for visualization.

ENDOSCOPIC RESECTION

The endoscopic approach for OGMs is the most recent development in surgical resection. It is generally performed by a neurosurgeon and an otorhinolaryngologist. The procedure is performed binaurally with the endoscope inserted through one nostril and the operating instruments through the opposite nostril. The procedure begins with bilateral maxillary antrostomies, complete ethmoidectomies and sphenoidotomies, as well as frontal sinusotomies. During this initial exposure, unilateral or bilateral nasoseptal flaps are harvested depending on the size of the anticipated defect. They are tucked into the maxillary sinus or nasopharynx during the course of the dissection. Once a standard bilateral endoscopic sinus surgery and nasoseptal flaps are harvested, a modified Lothrop procedure is performed. Special attention is given to removing the complete frontal intersinus septum and the nasal septum providing wide field of exposure for the dissection from the posterior wall of the frontal sinus to the anterior wall of the pituitary fossa.

During dissection, it is important to control the blood supply to the OGM. Bilateral anterior ethmoidal arteries are identified and ligated. In addition, the posterior ethmoid arteries are drilled out. Through image guidance, the anterior and posterior aspect of the OGM is identified. The anterior cut is generally made at the level of the posterior wall of the frontal sinus and continued along the fovea ethmoidalis using a combination of high-speed drill and Kerrison punches. The posterior resection is made as posterior as necessary given the size of the OGM. It can be made posteriorly to the planum sphenoidale, if necessary (**Fig. 3**).

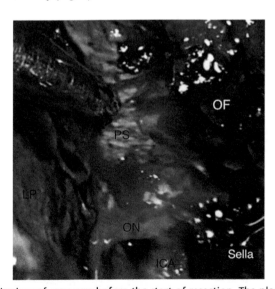

Fig. 3. Endoscopic view of exposure before the start of resection. The planum sphenoidale and cribriform plate have been resected. ICA, internal carotid artery at the parasellar carotid protuberance; LP, lamina paprycea; OF, olfactory filaments; ON, optic nerve; PS, planum sphenoidale; Sella, tuberculum sellae.

Next, the dura is incised exposing the entire OGM (**Fig. 4**). Resection of the OGM is completed in conjunction with the neurosurgical team using image guidance to identify the tumor margins. The resection is completed with a combination of microdebrider, suction, bipolar cautery, and blunt dissection. It is critical during resection to use neurosurgical techniques. We use suction in one hand to provide a clear field and provide traction of the tumor during dissection. In the other hand, we use blunt and sharp bayoneted dissectors in combination with debriding instruments such as the Nico Myriad and the Cavitron Ultrasonic Surgical Aspirator. We have not found the need to use specific frontal sinus instruments during dissection, primarily because the approach provides such a wide field of view with the sphenoidotomy, ethmoidectomy, and superior septectomy. The plane between the OGM and the arachnoid tissue is identified and the neoplasm is then resected. Care is taken to dissect this tumor-arachnoid plane. Frequently, the branches of the anterior cerebral arteries are encountered in the interhemispheric cleft.

Tumors that extend laterally past a vertical plane through the medial orbital wall may be considered suboptimal for an endoscopic resection because the medial orbital wall limits access intracranially. Although access is an issue with large tumors extending laterally, it is often possible to internally debulk the lateral aspect of the OGM and draw it toward the midline. Generally, we are able to completely excise tumors extending approximately 1 cm past the plane of the medial orbital wall.

The skull base defect is repaired initially with autologous fat graft. This repair is followed in an inlay fashion with either fascia lata or placement of Duragen (Integra Life Sciences, Boston, MA). After a watertight seal has been created, a thin layer of fibrin glue is applied at the edges of the defect. At this point, the nasoseptal flap is placed in an onlay fashion to cover the defect. Once lying flush, fibrin glue is again applied to the edges of the flap providing a "gasket" type closure. This repair is subsequently supported by nasal packing, which is positioned flush against the repair. The packing is generally left in place for 2 weeks.

The main advantage of the endoscopic approach compared with the previously described open approaches is the lack of brain retraction. This is a theoretic advantage because it is less significant for OGM compared with tuberculum sella

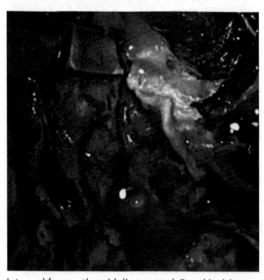

Fig. 4. Cribriform plate and fovea ethmoidalis resected. Dural incision made to expose OGM.

meningiomas, because OGM by definition are located more anteriorly and the overall retraction from open approaches is less. Nevertheless, we have seen a remarkable contrast between patients who undergo craniotomy versus endoscopic resection in the immediate postoperative period with respect to patient alertness, cognitive function, and overall ability to resume presurgical daily activities. This has not been shown in scientific study; it simply represents our experience.

Another critical advantage to the endoscopic approach is that the main site of recurrence, the anterior fossa floor, is completely excised endoscopically. Obeid and colleagues[37] suggested that recurrence of OGM is related to the gentle handling of the olfactory groove during craniotomy approaches. Obeid and colleagues[37] recommended that hyperostotic bone of the olfactory groove must be drilled out to minimize recurrence. In the endoscopic approach, resection of this area is required during exposure of the OGM and should help minimize recurrence.

The endoscopic approach also allows for 2 surgeons to operate simultaneously, which helps keep a dry field while dissecting. This approach gives superior exposure that cannot be matched with a craniotomy approach. The ability to keep a dry field, in combination with angled endoscopes, allows an improved view around edges of dura, enabling more complete resection and visualization of tumor borders. From a cosmetic standpoint, the endoscopic approach also provides outcomes that are superior to those of traditional craniotomy approaches.

Patient selection is critical to a successful outcome with an endoscopic approach. The biggest disadvantage to endoscopic resection of OGM is the risk for CSF leak. The overall leak rate with endoscopic resection is now less than 10%[38] because of evolving techniques in endoscopic reconstruction. The most recent advance in this area has been the advent of the posterior nasal septal mucosal flap.[39] The flap is pedicled on the posterior nasal septal artery and can be rotated to cover large skull base defects. When necessary, bilateral flaps may be harvested for reconstruction. Because this flap maintains its blood supply, the mucosa tends to recover quickly and generally heals within 5 to 7 days, creating a watertight seal. OGMs in general do not open large CSF cisterns, and the risk of CSF leak is lower than for a resection of a craniopharyngioma, for example. Nevertheless, we repair the defect with an autologous graft, fascia lata, and a vascularized mucosal flap.

Empty nose syndrome is another concern regarding extensive endonasal tumor resection. With the large amount of paranasal sinus structures removed, the patient theoretically has the potential to develop symptoms including paradoxic nasal obstruction and patient inability to sense nasal airflow.[40] In our resections, we do not alter the inferior turbinates, and attempt to leave at least 1 middle turbinate intact. In addition, special care is maintained not to traumatize any mucosa not in the field of resection. In our experience, for both OGM and other skull base tumor resections, we have not experienced patients with this complication.

The endoscopic approach is a recent advance in resections of OGMs. Gardner and colleagues[38] reported on a series of 15 patients who underwent an endoscopic resection. They had 12 of 15 patients with planned complete or near-total resection. A total of 10 of 12 eventually had at least near-total resections (>95%). Of the remaining 2 patients, 1 had an intraoperative frontopolar arterial bleed managed endoscopically. This procedure was terminated early. The second patient had his resection terminated early secondary to poor visualization as a result of venous congestion and bleeding. The patient subsequently underwent a successful open subfrontal approach. At this point, there is not enough literature to ascertain recurrence after endoscopic resections. The previously described study has a limited follow-up period (12–48 months), but reported no recurrence during this interval.[38]

CASE PRESENTATION

We present a patient with an OGM to highlight the surgical options available. He is a 66-year-old man who presented with severe headaches associated with nausea and emesis. The headaches began suddenly 3 weeks before presentation and were constant. He reports no visual changes or loss of smell. Other medical problems include chronic renal insufficiency for which he is on the renal transplant list, congestive heart failure, hypertension, diabetes, coronary artery disease, and atrial fibrillation. On physical examination, he was neurologically intact with no visual field deficits. MRI, which is performed without gadolinium because of renal insufficiency, shows a 3.7-cm OGM (**Fig. 5**).

We discussed at length with the patient his options including surgical therapy as well as his nonsurgical options. Despite his multiple medical problems, this was a highly functional individual who was interested in curative therapy. We reviewed his surgical options highlighting the advantages and disadvantages of each approach, and ultimately elected to perform an endoscopic resection. Although he was highly functional, we could not overlook his multiple comorbidities. We believed that an endoscopic approach would avoid any manipulation/retraction of his frontal lobe and provide a less invasive approach to resection. He ultimately underwent a complete endonasal resection and a reconstruction, which included a fat graft, fascia lata graft, and a pedicled nasoseptal flap. He had no complications from the procedure with no evidence of residual disease or recurrence (**Fig. 6**).

RT FOR MENINGIOMA

Although surgery is the only definitive option for OGMs, RT is indicated in certain situations. Tumors that have been incompletely excised often undergo radiation for residual tumor. In addition, atypical and malignant OGMs have a high recurrence rate even after complete gross resection. RT is routinely used in these situations as adjuvant therapy, although some data suggest that it may not be required after total resection of atypical OGMs.[5] RT may be used in cases of recurrence if not amendable to reresection.

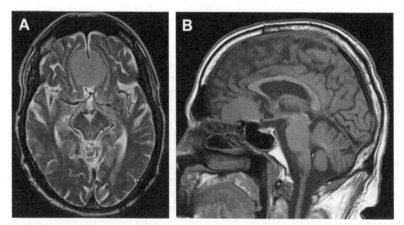

Fig. 5. (*A*) T2-weighted axial MRI of patient with OGM. Because of the patient's renal insufficiency, this scan was performed without gadolinium. (*B*) T1-weighted sagittal MRI without gadolinium of the same patient. Note that the posterior aspect of the OGM extends into the planum sphenoidale.

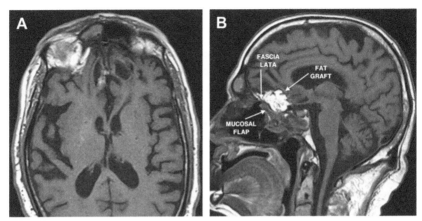

Fig. 6. (*A*) Posttreatment T1-weighted MRI showing complete resection of OGM. (*B*) Early posttreatment sagittal T1-weighted MRI without gadolinium. The reconstruction including the nasoseptal flap, fascia lata, and intracranial fat are in place. No evidence of residual disease.

SRS FOR MENINGIOMAS

SRS involves using multiple convergent external radiation beams to deliver a high single dose of radiation to a discrete tumor volume. The advantage of SRS is that it produces a rapid decrease of dose at the edge of the neoplasm, resulting in minimal radiation doses to normal, nontarget tissue. Because meningiomas are generally small, well circumscribed, and easily identified on neuroimaging, they are often treated with SRS.[41,42]

To reduce toxicity, fractionated SRS has also been studied for use on meningiomas. The potential advantages of fractionated SRS include the ability to treat larger tumors and even those tumors that are in close proximity to critical intracranial structures.

Currently, no published studies have shown that fractionated SRS has improved outcomes compared with standard SRS in the treatment of meningiomas. In the only reported comparative analysis, there was no clear difference in local control, toxicity, and impact on neurologic function.[43] To date, no literature has examined the use of SRS or fractionated SRS in OGMs because they are generally accessible surgically. In addition, although there are limited data, potential malignant transformation of benign meningiomas following SRS has been reported.[44] This has been a subject of debate because many believe that malignant transformation may have been either caused by the natural evolution of those reported cases or potentially be secondary to biopsy of the area. Given the accessibility of OGMs as well as the aforementioned reasons, SRS and other therapies at this point are reserved for recurrences, residual tumors, or those patients unable to tolerate surgical therapy.

CHEMOTHERAPY FOR MENINGIOMAS

The role of chemotherapy in meningiomas has been limited. In general, it is reserved for the treatment of tumors that recur after surgery after maximal RT has been completed. There have been small clinical trials and case series evaluating chemotherapeutic agents in meningiomas. Most have found that they have minimal activity against these neoplasms.[43,45–48] Some of these studies suggest an intermittent period of disease stabilization with chemotherapy, but the data are difficult to interpret, because untreated meningiomas are generally slow growing. Hydroxyurea is being evaluated for treatment of meningiomas and shows some benefit in several small studies.[47] The significance of these studies is difficult to ascertain because many of the patients were subsequently treated with RT. Currently, phase 2 trials are underway evaluating the role of hydroxyurea in the treatment of meningiomas.[47]

TARGETED MOLECULAR THERAPY

As in all neoplastic studies, continued work on targeted molecular therapy continues to gain widespread support. Emerging data have identified aberrant expression of key signaling molecules in meningioma cells.[49] Several pathways including inhibitors of growth signaling factors, inhibitors of angiogenesis, and inhibitors of hormonal targets are currently being investigated.

Imatinib is an inhibitor of PDGFR, a key driver of cell proliferation in meningiomas. A phase 2 study conducted by the North American Brain Tumor Consortium evaluated several patients with benign, atypical, and malignant meningiomas.[50] Although treatment was generally well tolerated, they found minimal response. In vitro studies have shown improved response of imatinib in combination with other protease inhibitors and proapoptotic agents.[51] These studies are currently ongoing.

Angiogenesis inhibitors are also undergoing several trials in other forms of cancer including colon, rectum, lung, kidney, and liver.[52] Bevacizumab is a monoclonal antibody against VEGF, and sorafenib and sunitinib are both small-molecule inhibitors of the VEGF receptors (VEGFR). Meningiomas express both VEGF and VEGFR and the level of expression increases with tumor grade.[53] In addition to its function in angiogenesis, VEGF is an important mediator of vascular permeability that promotes peritumoral edema in meningiomas.[54,55] Currently, clinical trials of these angiogenesis inhibitors for meningiomas are ongoing.

As previously mentioned, 10% of meningiomas have been found to have estrogen receptors, and approximately two-thirds have been found to have progesterone and androgen receptors. Targeted hormonal inhibitors are currently being investigated. Consistent with infrequent estrogen receptor expression, antiestrogen agents have not shown activity against meningiomas.[56] Initially there were some promising studies evaluating the antiprogesterone mifepristone (RU486), but in a randomized phase 3 study it showed no evidence of efficacy.[57] Androgen inhibitors have not been evaluated yet in meningioma therapy.

PROGNOSIS OF MENINGIOMA

When OGM resection results were initially reported, mortality was from 17.3% to 22.7%.[4,58] Recent literature has reduced mortality to nearly 0%.[35] At the current time, debate is centered on the optimal resection approach. Multiple factors including complete resection, brain retraction, CSF leak, potential for vascular injury, and size of the OGM contribute to decision making on approaches.

SUMMARY

Much has been reported on meningiomas because of their frequency. Currently, surgical resection is the mainstay of therapy. Similarly, OGMs are primarily treated surgically. Their unique location in the anterior cranial fossa adjacent to the skull base allows for a transnasal endoscopic resection of these tumors. To assess efficacy of endoscopic resection, continued long-term data are necessary. Alternative treatments are generally only used in the context of inoperable patients or unresectable recurrence.

Molecular targeted therapy continues to be an exciting and heavily researched aspect of meningioma therapy given the variety of potential targeting mechanisms.

EVIDENCE-BASED SUMMARY

Question: Is the morbidity of an endoscopic approach less than an open approach for OGM resection?

Answer: The key to OGM resection is understanding where the limitations are in an endoscopic approach. Endoscopically, the a complete resection of the hyperostotic bone of the olfactory groove is readily feasible. Conversely, an OGM with lateral extension much beyond the vertical plane of the medial orbital wall represents an endoscopic challenge and is better served with an open approach. Appropriate patient selection is critical in minimizing the morbidity of the respective procedures. In addition, the complications that arise are different for the endoscopic and open approaches.

The largest reported series of endoscopic resection of OGM is 15 by Gardner and colleagues.[38] Both the number and follow-up time (12–48 months) are too small a sample size to establish any evidence-based conclusions. What is clear is that postoperative CSF leaks seem to be the main complication in endoscopic resection. Gardner and colleagues[38] reported 4/15 (27%) posttreatment CSF leaks and all patients required revision CSF leak repair. Alternatively, open approaches report postoperative CSF leaks, but to a lesser extent.[32,34,59] In addition, reported series show that most CSF leaks in open cases can be managed with a lumbar drain alone.[32,34,59] These series have reported other complications such as intracranial hematoma, posttreatment seizures, increased frontal lobe edema, and other neurologic deficits. Aside from increased frontal lobe edema, presumably from brain retraction, all other complications are theoretically possible via an endoscopic approach, but have yet to be reported. Given the small sample size of endoscopic resections, with the largest series comprising 15, we cannot make any clear evidence-based statements.

Additional endoscopic data are necessary to definitively compare an open versus endoscopic approach. Furthermore, data sets such as duration of hospital stay, required rehabilitation, and Karnofsky scores will help to make an assessment of true postoperative morbidity. At this point, it is known that the type of complication will be based on the modality of resection, but, ultimately, despite both the theoretic advantages of an endoscopic approach and our anecdotal observation of decreased morbidity, we cannot make any evidence-based statement on postoperative morbidity of the endoscopic versus open approach for OGM resection.

EBM Question	Author's reply
Is the morbidity of an endoscopic approach less than an open approach for OGM resection?	CSF leak rates have reduced in recent years to be comparable to open surgery but although the inherent avoidance of craniotomy and frontal lobe retraction. There is no evidence to favour endoscopic or open surgery. Endoscopic removal of OGM with lateral extension much beyond the vertical plane of the medial orbital wall is very limited.

REFERENCES

1. Derome PJ, Guiot G. Bone problems in meningiomas invading the base of the skull. Clin Neurosurg 1978;25:435–51.

2. McDermott MW, Wilson CB. Meningiomas. 4th edition. Philadelphia: Saunders; 1996.
3. Hallacq P, Moreau JJ, Fischer G, et al. Trans-sinusal frontal approach for olfactory groove meningiomas. Skull Base 2001;11(1):35–46.
4. Cushing H, Eisenhardt L. The olfactory groove meningiomas with primary anosmia. In: Meningiomas: their classification, regional behavior, life history and surgical end results. Springfield (MA): Charles C Thomas; 1938. p. 250–73.
5. Goyal LK, Suh JH, Mohan DS, et al. Local control and overall survival in atypical meningioma: a retrospective study. Int J Radiat Oncol Biol Phys 2000;46(1):57–61.
6. Hentschel SJ, DeMonte F. Olfactory groove meningiomas. Neurosurg Focus 2003;14(6):e4.
7. Rowland LP, Pedley TA. Merritt's neurology. Philadelphia: Lippincott Williams & Wilkins; 2009.
8. Norden AD, Drappatx J, Wen PY. Advances in meningioma therapy. Curr Neurol Neurosci Rep 2009;9(3):231–40.
9. Louis DN, Budka H, von Deimling A, et al. In: Kielhues P, Cavenee WK, editors. World Health Organization classification of tumours. Pathology and genetics of tumours of the nervous system. Lyon (France): IARC Press; 2000. p. 176–84.
10. Lee JY, Finkelstein S, Hamilton RL, et al. Loss of heterozygosity analysis of benign, atypical, and anaplastic meningiomas. Neurosurgery 2004;55(5):1163–73.
11. Shen Y, Nunes F, Stemmer-Rachamimov A, et al. Genomic profiling distinguishes familial multiple and sporadic multiple meningiomas. BMC Med Genomics 2009; 2:42.
12. Hansson CM, Buckley PG, Grigelioniene G, et al. Comprehensive genetic and epigenetic analysis of sporadic meningioma for macro-mutations on 22q and micro-mutations within the NF2 locus. BMC Genomics 2007;8:16.
13. Ragel BT, Jensen RL. Molecular genetics of meningiomas. Neurosurg Focus 2005;19(5):E9.
14. Lee Y, Liu J, Patel S, et al. Genomic landscape of meningiomas. Brain Pathol 2010; 20(4):751–62.
15. Riemenschneider MJ, Perry A, Reifenberger G. Histological classification and molecular genetics of meningiomas. Lancet Neurol 2006;5(12):1045–54.
16. Hijiya N, Hudson MM, Lensing S, et al. Cumulative incidence of secondary neoplasms as a first event after childhood acute lymphoblastic leukemia. JAMA 2007;297(11):1207–15.
17. Preston DL, Ron E, Yonehara S, et al. Tumors of the nervous system and pituitary gland associated with atomic bomb radiation exposure. J Natl Cancer Inst 2002; 94(20):1555–63.
18. Ron E, Modan B, Bolce JD Jr, et al. Tumors of the brain and nervous system after radiotherapy in childhood. N Engl J Med 1988;319(16):1033–9.
19. Sadetzki S, Flint-Richter P, Starinsky S, et al. Genotyping of patients with sporadic and radiation-associated meningiomas. Cancer Epidemiol Biomarkers Prev 2005;14(4):969–76.
20. Sadetzki S, Flint-Richeter P, Ben-Tai T, et al. Radiation-induced meningioma: a descriptive study of 253 cases. J Neurosurg 2002;97(5):1078–82.
21. Wiemels J, Wrensch M, Claus EB. Epidemiology and etiology of meningioma. J Neurooncol 2010;99(3):307–14.
22. Claus EB, Black PM, Bondy ML, et al. Exogenous hormone use and meningioma risk: what do we tell our patients? Cancer 2007;110(3):471–6.
23. Vadivelu S, Sharer L, Schulder M. Regression of multiple intracranial meningiomas after cessation of long-term progesterone agonist therapy. J Neurosurg 2010;112(5):920–4.

24. Phillips LE, Koepseil TD, Van Belle G, et al. History of head trauma and risk of intracranial meningioma: population-based case-control study. Neurology 2002; 58(12):1849–52.
25. Preston-Martin S, Paganini-Hill A, Henderson BE, et al. Case-control study of intracranial meningiomas in women in Los Angeles County, California. J Natl Cancer Inst 1980;65(1):67–73.
26. Annegers JF, Laws ER Jr, Kurland LT, et al. Head trauma and subsequent brain tumors. Neurosurgery 1979;4(3):203–6.
27. Eskandary H, Sabba M, Khajehpur F, et al. Incidental findings in brain computed tomography scans of 3000 head trauma patients. Surg Neurol 2005;63(6):550–3 [discussion: 553].
28. Brenner AV, Linet MS, Fine HA, et al. History of allergies and autoimmune diseases and risk of brain tumors in adults. Int J Cancer 2002;99(2):252–9.
29. Krampla W, Newrkia S, Pfisterer W, et al. Frequency and risk factors for meningioma in clinically healthy 75-year-old patients: results of the Transdanube Ageing Study (VITA). Cancer 2004;100(6):1208–12.
30. Vernooij MW, Ikram MA, Tanghe HL, et al. Incidental findings on brain MRI in the general population. N Engl J Med 2007;357(18):1821–8.
31. Bakay L, Cares HL. Olfactory meningiomas. Report on a series of twenty-five cases. Acta Neurochir (Wien) 1972;26(1):1–12.
32. Tsikoudas A, Martin-Hirsch DP. Olfactory groove meningiomas. Clin Otolaryngol Allied Sci 1999;24(6):507–9.
33. DeMonte F. Surgical treatment of anterior basal meningiomas. J Neurooncol 1996;29(3):239–48.
34. Spektor S, Valarezo J, Fliss DM, et al. Olfactory groove meningiomas from neurosurgical and ear, nose, and throat perspectives: approaches, techniques, and outcomes. Neurosurgery 2005;57(Suppl 4):268–80 [discussion: 268–80].
35. Turazzi S, Cristofori L, Gambin R, et al. The pterional approach for the microsurgical removal of olfactory groove meningiomas. Neurosurgery 1999;45(4):821–5 [discussion: 825–6].
36. Hassler W, Zentner J. Pterional approach for surgical treatment of olfactory groove meningiomas. Neurosurgery 1989;25(6):942–5 [discussion 945–7].
37. Obeid F, Al-Mefty O. Recurrence of olfactory groove meningiomas. Neurosurgery 2003;53(3):534–42 [discussion: 542–3].
38. Gardner PA, Kassam AB, Thomas A, et al. Endoscopic endonasal resection of anterior cranial base meningiomas. Neurosurgery 2008;63(1):36–52 [discussion: 52–4].
39. Hadad G, Bassagastegy L, Carrau RL, et al. A novel reconstructive technique after endoscopic expanded endonasal approaches: vascular pedicle nasoseptal flap. Laryngoscope 2006;116(10):1882–6.
40. Chhabra N, Houser SM. The diagnosis and management of empty nose syndrome. Otolaryngol Clin North Am 2009;42(2):311–30, ix.
41. Lee JY, Niranjan A, McInerney J, et al. Stereotactic radiosurgery providing long-term tumor control of cavernous sinus meningiomas. J Neurosurg 2002;97(1):65–72.
42. Harris AE, Lee JY, Omalu B, et al. The effect of radiosurgery during management of aggressive meningiomas. Surg Neurol 2003;60(4):298–305 [discussion: 305].
43. Torres RC, Frighetto L, De Salles AA, et al. Radiosurgery and stereotactic radiotherapy for intracranial meningiomas. Neurosurg Focus 2003;14(5):e5.
44. Kubo O, Chernov M, Izawa M, et al. Malignant progression of benign brain tumors after gamma knife radiosurgery: is it really caused by irradiation? Minim Invasive Neurosurg 2005;48(6):334–9.

45. Chamberlain MC, Tsao-Wei DD, Groshen S. Temozolomide for treatment-resistant recurrent meningioma. Neurology 2004;62(7):1210–2.
46. Chamberlain MC, Tsao-Wei DD, Groshen S. Salvage chemotherapy with CPT-11 for recurrent meningioma. J Neurooncol 2006;78(3):271–6.
47. Newton HB. Hydroxyurea chemotherapy in the treatment of meningiomas. Neurosurg Focus 2007;23(4):E11.
48. Chamberlain MC, Glantz MJ, Fadul CE. Recurrent meningioma: salvage therapy with long-acting somatostatin analogue. Neurology 2007;69(10):969–73.
49. Simon M, Bostrom JP, Hartmann C. Molecular genetics of meningiomas: from basic research to potential clinical applications. Neurosurgery 2007;60(5): 787–98 [discussion: 787–98].
50. Wen PY, Drappatz J. Novel therapies for meningiomas. Expert Rev Neurother 2006;6(10):1447–64.
51. Gupta V, Samuleson CG, Su S, et al. Nelfinavir potentiation of imatinib cytotoxicity in meningioma cells via survivin inhibition. Neurosurg Focus 2007;23(4):E9.
52. Kerbel RS. Tumor angiogenesis. N Engl J Med 2008;358(19):2039–49.
53. Lamszus K, Lengler U, Schmidt NO, et al. Vascular endothelial growth factor, hepatocyte growth factor/scatter factor, basic fibroblast growth factor, and placenta growth factor in human meningiomas and their relation to angiogenesis and malignancy. Neurosurgery 2000;46(4):938–47 [discussion: 947–8].
54. Kan P, Liu JK, Wendland MM, et al. Peritumoral edema after stereotactic radiosurgery for intracranial meningiomas and molecular factors that predict its development. J Neurooncol 2007;83(1):33–8.
55. Provias J, Claffey K, Del Aguila L, et al. Meningiomas: role of vascular endothelial growth factor/vascular permeability factor in angiogenesis and peritumoral edema. Neurosurgery 1997;40(5):1016–26.
56. Goodwin JW, Crowley J, Eyre HJ, et al. A phase II evaluation of tamoxifen in unresectable or refractory meningiomas: a Southwest Oncology Group study. J Neurooncol 1993;15(1):75–7.
57. Grunberg SM, Rankin C, Townsend J, et al. Phase III double-blind randomized placebo-controlled study of mifepristone (RU) for the treatment of unresectable meningioma [abstract]. Proc ASCO 2001;20:222.
58. Solero CL, Giombini S, Morello G. Suprasellar and olfactory meningiomas. Report on a series of 153 personal cases. Acta Neurochir (Wien) 1983;67(3–4):181–94.
59. Tuna H, Bozkurt M, Ayten M, et al. Olfactory groove meningiomas. J Clin Neurosci 2005;12(6):664–8.
60. Lamszus K. Meningioma pathology, genetics, and biology. J Neuropathol Exp Neurol 2004;63:275–86.
61. Black PM, Morokoff AP, Zauberman J. Surgery for extra-axial tumors of the cerebral convexity and midline. Neurosurgery 2008;62:1115–21 [discussion: 1121–3].
62. Jaaskelainen J. Seemingly complete removal of histologically benign intracranial meningioma: late recurrence rate and factors predicting recurrence in 657 patients. A multivariate analysis. Surg Neurol 1986;26:461–9.
63. Yang SY, Park CK, Park SH, et al. Atypical and anaplastic meningiomas: prognostic implications of clinicopathological features. J Neurol Neurosurg Psychiatry 2008;79:574–80.

Endoscopic Endonasal Surgery for Nasal Dermoids

Carlos D. Pinheiro-Neto, MD[a], Carl H. Snyderman, MD, MBA[a,b,*],
Juan Fernandez-Miranda, MD[b], Paul A. Gardner, MD[b]

KEYWORDS

• Nasal dermoid • Skull base • Endoscopic endonasal approach

EBM Question	Level of Evidence	Grade of Recommendation
Is a craniotomy necessary to treat the intracranial component of a nasal dermoid?	5	D

Midline congenital lesions are rare and commonly comprise nasal dermoids (NDs), encephaloceles and gliomas. Among those lesions, NDs are the most common and account for 61% of midline nasal masses in children.[1] In 1817, Cruvelier described the first ND in a patient with a hair-containing sinus of the medial dorsal nose that had been present since birth.[2]

The incidence is estimated at 1 case per 20000 to 40000 births.[3,4] NDs account for 3.7% to 12.6% of all dermoids in the head and neck and 1% of all dermoid cysts through the body.[5,6] In literature, the incidence of intracranial extension of dermoids varies from 5% to 45%.[7–9] Males are slightly more affected than females.[7,10] Craniofacial abnormalities such as hypertelorism, hemifacial microsomia, cleft lip and/or palate, and craniosynostosis have been associated with NDs.[11]

PATHOPHYSIOLOGY

In 1910, Grunwald described a theory for ND formation. Embryogenesis of the midface occurs between 4 and 8 weeks of gestation. At the end of that process, a protrusion of

The authors have nothing to disclose.
[a] Department of Otolaryngology, University of Pittsburgh School of Medicine, 200 Lothrop Street, EEI Suite 500, Pittsburgh, PA 15213, USA
[b] Department of Neurological Surgery, University of Pittsburgh School of Medicine, 200 Lothrop Street, PUH 400, Pittsburgh, PA 15213, USA
* Corresponding author. Department of Otolaryngology, University of Pittsburgh School of Medicine, 200 Lothrop Street, EEI Suite 500, Pittsburgh, PA 15213.
E-mail address: snydermanch@upmc.edu

dura mater extends from the anterior cranial fossa through the foramen cecum to the space between the nasal bone and the deep layer of cartilaginous capsule (prenasal space). The dural diverticulum reaches and contacts the skin of the nasal tip. Subsequently, the fusion of the frontal and nasal bones occurs and the dural diverticulum involutes.

Failure during the regression of the dural diverticulum from the skin to the cranium results in a dermoid cyst or sinus. The contact of dura with the skin during embryogenesis may track skin elements from the nasal tip to the anterior cranial base. Proliferation of the trapped elements produces the typical lesion containing glands and hair. As the diverticulum courses from the cranial base to the tip of the nose, the ND can be extranasal, intranasal, intracranial, or a combination. Most commonly, NDs are restricted to the superficial nasal area. In case of intracranial extension, most often there is a communication through the foramen cecum to the anterior cranial base with extradural adherence to the falx.[12]

CLINICAL

NDs usually present at birth or in early childhood with a cosmetic deformity of the midface. Adult cases have also been reported. Typically it is a midline mass and may be situated from the collumella to the glabella. Sixty percent are located on the lower nasal dorsum; 30% are intranasal, and 10% are combined.[13]

NDs are typically a noncompressible mass and often present with nasal swelling or inflammation associated with a midline pit. Commonly, they end in a single subcutaneous tract with hair at the skin aperture. The presence of hair arising from the skin punctum is pathognomonic of ND.[11] Rarely, multiple ostia are present, and midline cysts may exist at more than 1 level.[2] Intermittent discharge of sebaceous material or pus when infected may be noticed.

Infection complications may occur as recurrent septum abscess and/or osteomyelitis.[13] The tract communicating with the anterior cranial base creates a potential risk for infection to spread intracranially. The patient may present with meningitis or brain abscess.[14]

Differential diagnosis for midline masses includes meningoencephaloceles and gliomas. Meningoencephaloceles consist of herniation of dura mater, cerebrospinal fluid (CSF), and brain matter through a bony defect. Gliomas are characterized by the presence of brain matter extracranially without dural connection. Because of those differences, encephaloceles typically enlarge with increases in intracranial pressure (Furstenburg sign), while gliomas and NDs do not change.[15] Meningoencephaloceles are usually softer and may transilluminate. Unlike NDs, gliomas do not contain skin elements (sebaceous gland secretions and hair). Besides those clinical differences, some lesions may only be differentiated with an adequate investigation.

INVESTIGATION

In case of clinical suspicious of ND, radiological imaging is essential to evaluate possible intracranial extension. Magnetic resonance imaging (MRI) seems to be superior compared with computed tomography (CT) scan for evaluation of intracranial extension.[16] However, the combination of both examinations is more precise for a good operative planning. The cuts should be planned to evaluate the entire frontoglabellar region. The use of contrast is valuable to differentiate enhancing nasal mucosa or lesions (hemangiomas/teratomas) from nonenhancing dermoid cysts.[17]

Typically, CT scan shows an enlarged foramen cecum and a bifid crista galli, which are suggestive of intracranial involvement.[18] However, some authors have published that the presence of those findings are not pathognomonic of intracranial extension. The presence of fibrous tissue connecting the dermoid cyst to the dura may provoke an enlarged foramen cecum and bifid crista galli without true intracranial extension of the cyst.[19] MRI is better to analyze soft tissue and consequent presence of intracranial involvement. It is important to note that the crista galli in infants is not ossified, and a high-intensity signal on T1-weighted images in that region should suggest intracranial dermoid.[20]

Nasal endoscopy should be part of the investigation for ND. Nasal endoscopy is usually normal in ND with an extranasal mass. Intranasal lesions may present as a septal submucosal mass protruding from both sides of the septum. The nasal endoscopy is also helpful for the assessment of the degree of nasal obstruction caused by the mass and impact on sinus drainage.

MANAGEMENT OF NDs

The treatment of ND is surgical resection. Radiation therapy and chemotherapy are not recommended in the management of these lesions.[21] The goal of surgery is complete resection of the cyst and its tract. Failure to achieve a complete resection of the tract may result in recurrence. Reports in literature vary from 50% to 100% recurrence rate when the cyst/tract elements are not completely resected.[16,22]

Several external approaches have been described for the treatment of ND (bicoronal or transfacial approaches). As an advantage, these approaches are sufficient to guarantee an adequate resection of extranasal, intranasal, and intracranial lesions. However, they have significant disadvantages: skin scar, alopecia (bicoronal), and brain retraction.

Recently, endoscopic approaches to treat ND have been published. The main advantages are good visualization, better cosmetic results, and avoidance of brain retraction for intracranial lesions. The endoscopic approach to ND can use the nasal cavity as a corridor (endoscopic endonasal) or subcutaneous tunnels through small incisions in the scalp, eyelid, or columella (endoscopic-assisted approaches).

PROGNOSIS AND NATURAL HISTORY

With incomplete resection, recurrence is common. Patients can present with episodes of cellulitis, nasal abscess, osteomyelitis, meningitis, or brain abscess. Untreated intracranial lesions may grow and cause intracranial hypertension or hydrocephalus. Intracranial infectious complications can lead to death if the lesion is not treated correctly or left untreated.

EVIDENCE-BASED MEDICINE REVIEW

There is a lack of literature regarding endoscopic treatment of ND. Most papers are case reports and have focused on endoscopic-assisted approaches using external incisions for lesions without intracranial extension. The number of papers published about endoscopic resection of ND with intracranial extension is even more limited (**Table 1**).

Lachica published a case of a patient with a nasoglabellar dermoid treated with an endoscopic-assisted surgery. With a small incision in the hairline, he dissected the forehead in a subperiosteal plane until reaching the nasoglabellar region. Using that approach, the author was able to resect the entire cyst. After 1 year of follow-up, the patient was satisfied with the result and with no evidence of recurrence.[23]

Lee published 2 cases of patients successfully treated with endoscopic-assisted surgery for nasoglabellar dermoid. One of them had an incision done in the hairline and the other one, in a crease of the upper eyelid.[24]

Table 1
Literature review of endoscopic treatment for nasal dermoids

Author	Number of Patients	Approach	Intracranial Extension	Complete Resection	Notes
Lachica et al,[23] 2004	1	Endoscopic-assisted (hairline incision)	No	Yes	1 year follow-up; no recurrence
Lee et al,[24] 2010	2	Endoscopic-assisted (1 patient with a hairline incision and the other with a upper eyelid incision)	No	Yes	
Weiss et al,[25] 1998	2	Endoscopic endonasal associated with excision of skin punctum	Yes	Yes	No intraoperative cerebrospinal fluid leak
Duz et al,[26] 2004	1	Endoscopic endonasal	Yes	Yes	Reconstruction with fascia lata and middle turbinate pedicled flap; 6 months follow-up; no recurrence
Schuster et al,[27] 2011	2	Endoscopic endonasal	Yes	Yes	Nasoseptal flap for reconstruction

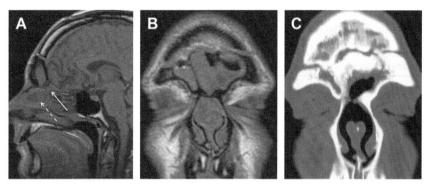

Fig. 1. 13-year-old boy presenting with recurrence of a nasal dermoid with intracranial extension. The patient was treated previously with a craniotomy by another service. (*A*) Magnetic resonance imaging (MRI) T1 without contrast sagittal view. Note the lesion in the nasal septum (*dashed arrow*) and the intracranial extension through the foramen cecum (*white arrow*). (*B*) MRI T1 without contrast coronal view. Note the lesion involving the nasal septum. (*C*) Postoperative computed tomography (CT) scan coronal view. Complete removal of the tumor after endoscopic endonasal surgery. Note frontal bone defect from previous craniotomy.

Considering the endoscopic endonasal approach for resection of intracranial ND, there are few cases described in the literature. In 1998, Weiss successfully treated 2 patients with ND with intracranial extension using a transnasal endoscopic approach. The authors suggested that endoscopic endonasal surgery is feasible when the lesion is located within the nasal cavity, and there is minimal or no cutaneous involvement. In cases where the skin is compromised, the endoscopic approach can be combined with a short vertical midline lenticular excision of the cutaneous punctum. From the skin incision, the resection of the tract should be done until communication with the lesion dissected endonasally. It is important to notice that in his series, all lesions had intracranial extension but were not intradural. There was a fibrous connection tissue between the lesion and the dura. In those 2 cases, no CSF leak was observed intraoperatively.[25]

In 2004, Duz presented a case of a patient with intradural dermoid who was treated with fully endoscopic endonasal approach. He achieved total gross resection in a piece-meal fashion. Dural reconstruction was done with fascia lata and middle turbinate pedicled flap. The patient was symptom-free at 6 months of follow up.[26]

In 2011, Schuster reported successful endoscopic resection of 2 intracranial dermoids with large anterior frontal lobe extensions, using a 70° endoscope and a pedicled nasoseptal flap to close the skull base defect.[27]

SUMMARY

Considering the evolution of endoscopic endonasal approaches for skull base lesions observed in the last decade, it is natural to question whether those approaches could be applied to treat ND. Literature review demonstrates minimal data regarding endoscopic endonasal resection of intracranial dermoids. The initial experience is supportive, however, and experience with endoscopic endonasal approaches for other pathologies in the same region suggests that the same techniques can be applied for intracranial extension of ND when performed by experienced endoscopic surgeons (**Fig. 1**).

EBM Question	Author's reply
Is a craniotomy necessary to treat the intracranial component of a nasal dermoid?	Case reports demonstrate that intracranial dermoids can be removed endoscopically but should be performed by experienced endoscopic surgeons.

REFERENCES

1. Rohrich RJ, Lowe JB, Schwartz MR. The role of open rhinoplasty in the management of nasal dermoid cysts. Plast Reconstr Surg 1999;104:2163–70.
2. Sessions RB. Nasal dermal sinuses: new concepts and explanations. Laryngoscope 1982;92(Suppl 29):1–28.
3. Pratt LW. Midline cysts of the nasal dorsum: embryologic origin and treatment. Laryngoscope 1965;75:968–80.
4. Hughes GB, Sharpino G, Hunt W, et al. Management of the congenital midline nasal mass: a review. Head Neck Surg 1980;2(3):222–33.
5. Crawford JK, Webster JP. Congenital dermoid cysts of the nose. Plast Reconstr Surg 1952;9:235–60.
6. New GB, Erich JB. Dermoid cysts of the head and neck. Surg Gynecol Obstet 1937;65:48–55.
7. Rahbar R, Shah P, Mulliken JB, et al. The presentation and management of nasal dermoid: a 30-year experience. Arch Otolaryngol Head Neck Surg 2003;129: 464–71.
8. Vaghela HM, Bradley PJ. Nasal dermoid sinus cyst in adults. J Laryngol Otol 2004;118:955–62.
9. van Aalst JA, Luerssen TG, Whitehead WE, et al. Keystone approach for intracranial nasofrontal dermoid sinuses. Plast Reconstr Surg 2005;116(1):13–9.
10. Denoyelle F, Ducroz V, Roger G, et al. Nasal dermoid sinus cysts in children. Laryngoscope 1997;107:795–800.
11. Wardinsky TD, Pagon RA, Kropp RJ, et al. Nasal dermoid sinus cysts: association with intracranial extension and multiple malformations. Cleft palate Craniofac J 1991;28:87–95.
12. Grunwald L. Bettrage zur kenntnis kongenitaler geschwulste und missbildungen an ohf und nase. Ztsch F Ohrenhik 1910;60:270.
13. Szeremeta W, Parikh TD, Widelitz JS. Congenital nasal malformations [review]. Otolaryngol Clin North Am 2007;40:97–112, vi–vii.
14. Locke R, Kubba H. The external rhinoplasty approach for congenital nasal lesions in children. Int J Pediatr Otorhinolaryngol 2011;75(3):337–41.
15. Hanikeri M, Waterhouse N, Kirkpatrick N, et al. The management of midline transcranial nasal dermoid sinus cysts. Br J Plast Surg 2005;58(8):1043–50.
16. Bloom DC, Carvalho DS, Dory C, et al. Imaging and surgical approach of nasal dermoids. Int J Pediatr Otorhinolaryngol 2002;62:111–22.
17. Zapata S, Kearns DB. Nasal dermoids. Curr Opin Otolaryngol Head Neck Surg 2006;14(6):406–11.
18. Manning S, Bloom D, Perkins J, et al. Diagnostic and surgical challenges in the pediatric skull base. Otolaryngol Clin North Am 2005;38:773–94.
19. Penslar JM, Bauer BS, Naidich TP. Craniofacial dermoids. Plast Reconstr Surg 1988;82:953–9.
20. Fornadley JA, Tami TA. The use of magnetic resonance imaging in the diagnosis of the nasal dermal sinus–cyst. Otolaryngol Head Neck Surg 1989;101(3):397–8.

21. Conley FK. Epidermoid and dermoid tumors: clinical features and surgical management. In: Wilkins RH, Rengachary SS, editors. Neurosurgery. New York: McGraw-Hill; 1985. p. 668–73.
22. Posnick JC, Bortoluzzi P, Armstrong DC, et al. Intracranial nasal dermoid sinus cysts: computed tomographic scan findings and surgical results. Plast Reconstr Surg 1994;3:745–54.
23. Lachica RD, Wallace RD, Tsujimura RB. Case report: endoscopic excision of a nasoglabellar dermoid. J Craniofac Surg 2004;15(3):473–7.
24. Lee S, Taban M, Mancini R, et al. Endoscopic removal of nasoglabellar dermoid cysts. Ophthal Plast Reconstr Surg 2010;26(2):136–9.
25. Weiss DD, Robson CD, Mulliken JB. Transnasal endoscopic excision of midline nasal dermoid from the anterior cranial base. Plast Reconstr Surg 1998;102(6): 2119–23.
26. Düz B, Secer HI, Tosun F, et al. Endoscopic endonasal resection of a midline intradural frontobasal dermoid tumour. Minim Invasive Neurosurg 2007;50(6): 363–6.
27. Schuster D, Riley KO, Cure JK, et al. Endoscopic resection of intracranial dermoid cysts. J Laryngol Otol 2011;125(4):423–7.

Juvenile Nasopharyngeal Angiofibroma

Angela Blount, MD[a], Kristen O. Riley, MD[b],
Bradford A. Woodworth, MD[c],*

KEYWORDS

- Juvenile nasopharyngeal angiofibroma • Endoscopic surgery
- Embolization • Sinus surgery • Epistaxis • Sinonasal tumor
- Skull base tumor • Nasopharyngeal tumor

EBM Question	Level of Evidence	Grade of Recommendation
Is morbidity less with endoscopic resection (blood loss, cosmesis, CN injury, etc) compared to open surgery?	3b	C

SYMPTOMS OF JNA

The most common presenting symptoms of patients with JNA are unilateral nasal obstruction occurring in 91% and epistaxis occurring in 63% of patients.[2] Other related symptoms include nasal discharge; pain; sinusitis; facial deformity; otologic symptoms, such as hearing impairment and otitis media; and ocular symptoms of proptosis and diplopia.[2] Symptoms are generally present for 6 months to a year before the patient is diagnosed. JNAs are typically found in the male population between the ages of 10 and 24 years, with a median age at diagnosis of 15 years.[2]

Disclosure statement: Brad Woodworth MD is a consultant for Arthrocare ENT and Gyrus ENT.
[a] Division of Otolaryngology–Head and Neck Surgery, University of Alabama at Birmingham, 563 Boshell Building, 1530 3rd Avenue South, Birmingham, AL 35294-0012, USA
[b] Division of Neurological Surgery, University of Alabama at Birmingham, 1530 3rd Avenue South, Birmingham, AL 35294, USA
[c] Division of Otolaryngology–Head and Neck Surgery, Department of Surgery, University of Alabama at Birmingham, 563 Boshell Building, 1530 3rd Avenue South, Birmingham, AL 35294-0012, USA
* Corresponding author.
E-mail address: brad.woodworth@ccc.uab.edu

Key Points: JUVENILE NASOPHARYNGEAL ANGIOFIBROMA

- Endoscopic resection of early-stage juvenile nasopharyngeal angiofibromas (JNAs) is a safe and surgically sound treatment that has multiple advantages over traditional open approaches, including better cosmesis, decreased blood loss, shortened hospital stay, and equivalent or improved recurrence rates.

- Magnetic resonance imaging (MRI) is the imaging standard for postoperative surveillance and should be performed within the first postoperative year to detect recurrent/residual disease.

- First described by Chaveau in 1906,[1] JNAs are highly vascular benign tumors that primarily affect the young male population. These neoplasms are rare, accounting for approximately 0.05% of head and neck tumors. Although benign and slow growing, these tumors are locally aggressive and can cause extensive bone destruction, intracranial hemorrhage, facial deformity, severe epistaxis, and blindness. JNAs derive from the superior border of the sphenopalatine foramen. As the tumors enlarge, they extend through well-defined pathways into the infratemporal fossa, cavernous sinus, sphenoid sinus, middle cranial fossa, and, rarely, anterior cranial fossa. Surgical resection has been the mainstay of treatment of JNAs, and multiple open surgical approaches have been proposed depending on the location and extent of the tumor. Radiation therapy has been mostly reserved for unresectable tumors, residual disease after surgical resection, or recurrences occurring in anatomically critical areas. However, over the past 2 decades, endoscopic techniques and technology have improved, and an increasing number of JNAs are being removed endoscopically or in combination with traditional open approaches. Endoscopic techniques offer many advantages over open approaches, with better cosmesis (no external surgical scar), reduced intraoperative blood loss (usually combined with preoperative embolization), decreased hospital stays, and improved or equivalent recurrence rates.

PATHOLOGY OF JNA

JNAs are characterized on gross pathology as well-defined, mucosalized, red to purple masses found in the nasal cavity and nasopharynx (**Fig. 1**). Histologically, the tumor is composed of 2 main components: spindle- or stellate-shaped cells embedded in a rich collagen matrix and a complex vascular arrangement of blood vessels that vary in size from capillaries to large venous channels. Characteristically, these vessels lack elastic laminae and elastic fibers and have vascular walls that vary in thickness. These features account for the tendency of these tumors to hemorrhage easily.[3] JNAs occur exclusively in men and are thought to be partially androgen dependent. JNAs possess multiple hormone receptors, including testosterone, dihydrotestosterone, and androgen.[4] However, investigation into hormone therapy for these tumors has been disappointing. JNAs may originate from a residual vascular plexus left behind after the involution of the first branchial artery,[5] but the cause of JNAs is still under debate.

IMAGING

Computed tomography (CT) and MRI are both critical to the proper evaluation of angiofibromas. CT better delineates bony details of the skull base, including bony erosion, in particular, the depth of invasion into the bone of the sphenoid sinus, a main predictor of recurrence (**Fig. 2**). The extent of invasion into the cancellous bone of the sphenoid is difficult to determine intraoperatively, and this leads to a high likelihood of residual tumor and recurrence.[6,7] CT scans are also commonly used for intraoperative stereotactic surgical navigation systems to confirm the extent and resection of tumor. On the other hand, MRI is crucial for highlighting soft tissue

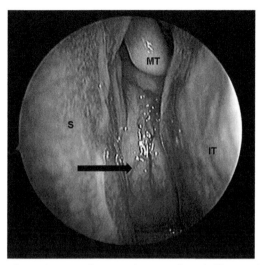

Fig. 1. Transnasal endoscopic view of a nasopharyngeal angiofibroma (*arrow*) in the right nasal cavity. IT, inferior turbinate; MT, middle turbinate; S, septum.

elements of the tumor and assesses the relation of the tumor to critical structures such as the internal carotid artery, cavernous sinus, and pituitary gland (**Fig. 3**). Recurrence and residual tumors are best appreciated on MRI.

The pathognomonic radiologic feature of JNAs is the anterior bowing of the posterior maxillary wall, termed the Holman-Miller sign. Other radiologic features include

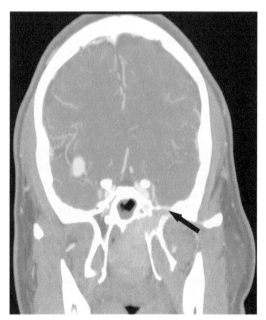

Fig. 2. Coronal CT angiogram demonstrating a large JNA filling the nasopharynx and eroding the middle cranial fossa skull base (*arrow*) via an extension of the tumor posterior to the left pterygoid plates. There was an incidental finding of a right cerebral aneurysm.

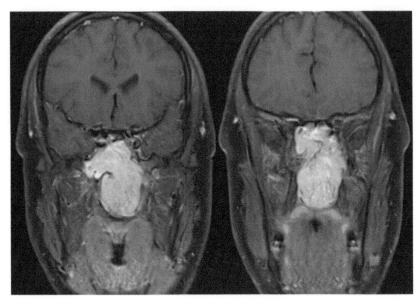

Fig. 3. Coronal MRI scan with gadolinium reveals a left-sided JNA with significant soft tissue enhancement. Note that the entire posterior nasal cavity, nasopharynx, and sphenoid sinuses are occupied bilaterally with tumor.

a mass originating at the sphenopalatine foramen and erosion of the mass into the pterygomaxillary fossa, sphenoid sinus, and infratemporal fossa.[6,8]

Further confirmation of the JNA diagnosis is usually provided by angiography, which also doubles as treatment with embolization. Angiography provides information on the specific blood supply of the tumor. Distal branches of the internal maxillary artery, a branch of the external carotid, provide the major blood supply for most JNAs, but, as tumors grow, they may also develop vascular supply from branches of the ipsilateral internal carotid artery and contralateral external carotid artery.[9,10] **Fig. 4** shows the extensive vascular network of a JNA as seen in reconstructed images from angiography and CT angiography.

STAGING FOR NASOPHARYNGEAL ANGIOFIBROMAS

Several staging systems for nasopharyngeal angiofibromas have been proposed, all based on extension of the tumor. The 3 most prevalent staging systems are those of Andrews' (modified Fisch),[11] Chandler's,[12] and Radkowski's[13] (modification of Sessions' classification). JNAs are classified depending on the extension of tumor and amount of intracranial extension.[11] At present, there is no single universally adopted classification system. To better interpret the results of this article, all 3 classification systems have been included in **Tables 1–3**. A recently proposed endoscopic staging system for angiofibromas by Snyderman and colleagues[14] focuses on residual vascularity (after preoperative embolization) and route of intracranial extension. This novel classification aims to better predict morbidity and prognosis by focusing on these 2 critical features.[14]

TREATMENT OPTIONS FOR JNA

Surgical resection is widely accepted as the treatment modality of choice for JNAs. Multiple surgical approaches have been proposed and are often based on tumor

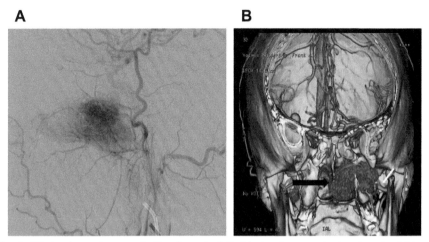

Fig. 4. (*A*) Angiography reveals the characteristic blush of a prevalent network of blood vessels within the JNA. (*B*) Three-dimensional reconstruction of a JNA (*black arrow*) from CT angiography. Note the extensive vascular network and the internal maxillary artery (*white arrow*), the main vascular supply for most of these tumors.

size, location, and extent. Recently, endoscopic approaches have been adopted, secondary to the likelihood of decreased morbidity. Adjunctive radiation, hormone therapy, and chemotherapy have all been explored, with hormone therapy and chemotherapy nearly abandoned because of ineffectiveness and significant side effects. However, radiation therapy is still widely used, although primarily saved for advanced tumors that would have a high morbidity with attempted resection or residual/recurrent disease in critical anatomic areas.[9,15] To complicate the issue of treatment, JNAs may spontaneously regress without any treatment once the patient completes adolescence. Spontaneous involution has been documented in multiple case reports.[16–19]

Radiation Therapy for JNA

Recent studies using radiation therapy as the definitive treatment of advanced JNAs have shown impressive local control rates of 85% to 91%. Reddy and colleagues[20]

Table 1	
Andrews' classification (modified Fisch) of JNAs	
Stage	**Description**
I	Tumor limited to the nasal cavity and nasopharynx
II	Tumor extension into the pterygopalatine fossa, maxillary, sphenoid, or ethmoid sinuses
IIIa	Extension into orbit or infratemporal fossa without intracranial extension
IIIb	Stage IIIa with small extradural intracranial (parasellar) involvement
IVa	Large extradural intracranial or intradural extension
IVb	Extension into cavernous sinus, pituitary, or optic chiasm

Data from Andrews JC, Fisch U, Valavanis A, et al. The surgical management of extensive nasopharyngeal angiofibromas with the infratemporal fossa approach. Laryngoscope 1989;99:429–37.

Table 2
Chandler's classification of JNAs

Stage	Description
I	Confined to nasopharynx
II	Extends into nasal cavity and/or sphenoid
III	Extends to 1 or several of the following: antrum, ethmoids, pterygomaxillary and infratemporal fossa, orbit, and/or cheek
IV	Extends into cranial cavity

Data from Chandler JR, Goulding R, Moskowitz L, et al. Nasopharyngeal angiofibromas: staging and management. Ann Otol Rhinol Laryngol 1984;93(4 Pt 1):322–9.

treated 15 patients with Chandler stage III or IV disease with 30 to 36 Gy of radiation, with a local control rate of 85%. Two patients with continued growth required further treatment with surgical salvage. The investigators also noted that tumor regression could take up to 2 years or more. An extension of this study treated 7 additional patients (reporting as a total of 22) and claimed a local control rate of 91% with no severe complications.[21] Lee and colleagues[22] treated 27 patients with 30 to 40 Gy, with 4 patients (15%) ultimately developing further growth requiring additional treatment. In the rest (85%), the tumor remained stable in size or regressed. However, the investigators did not consider radiographic abnormalities on imaging as residual or recurrent disease. Only if the patient became symptomatic or new radiographic findings developed was the condition considered to have recurred. Although rare, radiation may lead to devastating sequelae, including secondary head and neck malignancies, in this young population. Reddy and colleagues[20] had 1 patient who develop a basal cell carcinoma of the skin. Malignant transformation of the tumor with increasing radiation doses has also occurred in a small number of cases.[22] Other complications of radiation therapy include panhypopituitarism, growth retardation, cataracts, radiation keratopathy, temporal lobe necrosis, and delayed transient central nervous system syndrome.[20,22] Newer radiation techniques, such as intensity-modulated radiation therapy, may provide the same local control rates with less morbidity but are still under investigation for the treatment of JNAs.[23]

Table 3
Radkowski's classification (modification of Sessions' classification) of JNAs

Stage	Description
IA	Limited to nose and nasopharyngeal area
IB	Extension into 1 or more sinuses
IIA	Minimal extension into pterygopalatine fossa
IIB	Occupation of the pterygopalatine fossa with or without orbital erosion
IIC	Infratemporal fossa extension with or without cheek or pterygoid plate involvement
IIIA	Erosion of the skull base (middle cranial fossa or pterygoids)
IIIB	Erosion of skull base with intracranial extension with or without cavernous sinus involvement

Data from Radkowski D, McGill T, Healy GB, et al. Angiofibroma. Changes in staging and treatment. Arch Otolaryngol Head Neck Surg 1996;122:122–9.

Embolization

Before a debate on surgical techniques can begin, the issue of preoperative emboli-zation must be introduced. It is well accepted that preoperative embolization of JNAs significantly decreases blood loss during resection and improves visualization for more complete tumor removal.[24,25] Li and colleagues[26] found that operative blood loss in patients who underwent embolization was approximately half compared with those who did not undergo embolization (677 mL compared with 1136 mL). In addi-tion, in patients who did have a transfusion, those who underwent embolization re-quired only 400 mL of blood, whereas those who did not undergo embolization required 836 mL (a reduction of 50%). However, the significant risks of embolization cannot be discounted. These risks include, but are not limited to, neurologic deficits (numbness, facial paralysis), stroke, and blindness. Herman and colleagues[27] recently published a novel embolization technique with Onyx, a liquid embolic agent that is directly injected into the tumor under fluoroscopic and endoscopic guidance, that may prove to be safer and less invasive than traditional techniques. Some investiga-tors propose that preoperative embolization distorts tumor boundaries, leading to incomplete resection, especially if the tumor extends into the basisphenoid.[7] Lloyd[7] and Mann and colleagues[28] both suggest that preoperative embolization may increase recurrence rates secondary to incomplete tumor removal. Techniques to decrease bleeding without preoperative embolization have included hypotensive general anesthesia, with some reporting excellent results.[29] With novel technologies, such as radiofrequency coblation, tumors may be resected with significantly less blood loss,[30,31] and preoperative embolization may ultimately be deemed unneces-sary for lower-stage tumors. For example, Ruiz[32] has routinely used coblation for the resection of JNAs without preoperative embolization. Overall, however, in most endoscopic series, patients still undergo preoperative embolization 24 to 48 hours before surgery (significant contributions may develop from contralateral vessels several days after embolization).

Open Surgical Treatment of JNA

Multiple surgical approaches have been used for the resection of JNAs, including transpalatal, lateral rhinotomy, midface degloving, medial maxillectomy, transantral, infratemporal fossa, and frontotemporal craniotomy.[33,34] Different investigators recommend varied approaches, all dependent on the location and extension of the tumor. Before endoscopic approaches, the transpalatal and midface degloving approaches were popularized because they require no external surgical incisions.[24,34,35] Howard and colleagues[35] treated 19 cases of JNA with the midface degloving approach and reported no recurrences with 6 months to 3 years of follow-up. Tyagi and colleagues[33] used an extended transpalatal/transmaxillary approach for stage IIIa and IIIb disease (Andrews' classification) in 75 patients with a recurrence rate of 13%. The most common surgical complications were secretory otitis media and palatal fistulas. Hosseini and colleagues[36] used a transpalatal approach in 27 of 37 patients ranging from stage Ia to stage IIIb disease (Radkowski's classification), with 2 having residual disease and 4 patients developing recurrence. The most common postoperative compli-cation was oronasal fistula.

Endoscopic Resection

Endoscopic resection of benign and malignant neoplasms has gained significant ground in the past decade as a valuable alternative surgical approach.[37-39] Endo-scopic surgery has advantages over traditional open approaches, specifically in the male adolescent population that is affected by JNA. Endoscopic resection avoids osteotomies, which have been implicated in inhibiting facial growth.[40] This technique also requires no external incision or facial deforming scar, a concern in a population that is just beginning to develop their self-perception. In addition, endoscopes offer magnification and angled views for excellent tumor visualization not provided by open approaches.[41] Many investigators have detailed the feasibility of endoscopic approaches to early-stage JNAs.[34,41,42] However, controversy has abounded over which JNAs are most appropriate for endoscopic removal. Most investigators concede that early-stage JNAs (stage I, II, and some stage III) can be adequately removed endoscopically (**Figs. 5** and **6**).[41–43] Proponents of endoscopic resection report decreased length of hospital stays, reduced intraoperative blood loss, and equivalent or reduced recurrence rates compared with open approaches.

Blood loss

Bleier and colleagues[10] performed resection in 10 patients with stage I to stage IIIa disease (Andrews' classification) via a transnasal approach. The investigators reported that the endoscopic approach led to a 50% reduction in intraoperative blood loss compared with open approaches (both groups underwent preoperative embolization). Hackman and colleagues[44] reported a trend of reduced operative time and blood loss (280 mL vs 2500 mL) in endoscopic resection of JNAs compared with open approaches. Improved technology for hemostasis and other operative hemostatic appliances, such as radiofrequency coblation (see **Fig. 5B**), may improve endoscopic results by decreasing blood loss.[45]

Hospital stay

Andrade and colleagues[41] used exclusive endoscopic techniques to perform resection in 12 patients with stage I to II disease (Andrews'), resulting in a mean hospital stay of 33 hours for stage I disease and 54 hours for stage II disease. Bleier and colleagues[10] also reported decreased length of hospital stays with an average of 3 days in the endoscopic group and 4 days in the open group. Carrau and colleagues[43] described that patients with endoscopic resection were discharged the same or next day, whereas those who underwent open approaches remained in the hospital for up to 5 days. In short, most reductions in hospital stay may be attributed to the adoption of endoscopic techniques.

Endoscopic recurrence

General recurrence rates for JNA range from 13% to 46% depending on the literature.[8,10,28,33,35,46] Endoscopic recurrence rates have generally been lower, but this may be attributable to the bias that early-stage tumors are more likely to be treated endoscopically. Wormald and Hasselt[25] performed endoscopic resection in 7 patients with stage I to IIc disease (Radkowski's classification), with none developing recurrence after a mean follow-up of 3.75 years. Andrade and colleagues[41] also reported no recurrent or residual disease after a mean follow-up of 24 months in 12 patients with stage I to II disease (Andrew's classification). Borghei and colleagues[29] reported on 23 patients who underwent transnasal approach for JNA, all stage IA to IIB (Radkowski's classification), and only 1 patient (4.3%) developed a recurrence (19 months postoperatively original tumor stage IIB). Nicolai and colleagues[34] reported a rate of 8.6% for persistent disease for endoscopically removed JNAs staged I to IIIB (Andrews' classification), with a mean follow-up of 73 months. In general, endoscopic resection of JNAs has equivalent, if not better, recurrence rates compared with traditional open surgery.

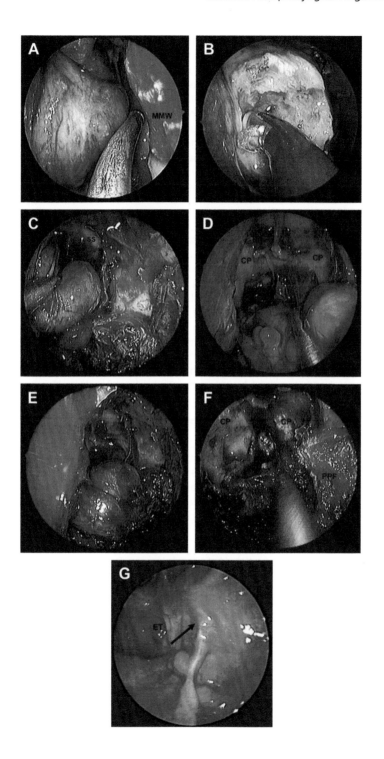

Complications with endoscopic resection

There have been few significant complications with endoscopic resection of JNAs. The most common complication for both open and endoscopic approaches is intraoperative hemorrhage, which, as discussed earlier, is decreased when using endoscopic techniques. Complications unique to endoscopy are few. Synechia formation in the nasal cavity seems to be the most common complication.[29] Carrau and colleagues[43] reported 1 case of optic neuropathy that resolved after prompt endoscopic decompression. Nicolai and colleagues[34] had no minor or major postoperative complications in 46 patients who underwent endoscopic resection of JNA. On the whole, endoscopic resection of JNAs in surgeons with appropriate training is a safe procedure with relatively few complications.

Limits of endoscopic resection

Endoscopic approaches coupled with frameless stereotactic image guidance continue to challenge the boundaries of resection, with some investigators advocating its use for advanced-stage tumors, including those with intracranial extension.[34] Because cerebrospinal fluid leaks can be successfully repaired endoscopically in most cases,[47–54] large skull base defects created by tumor removal are no longer a contraindication to endoscopic removal. As it stands, absolute contraindications to endoscopic approach with the intent of complete removal include encasement of the internal carotid artery, majority of the vascular supply from the internal carotid artery; significant involvement of the cavernous sinus; extensive intracranial extension; and lateral extension into the cheek.[28,34,42,55] Endoscopic techniques can be used successfully to remove early-stage and some later-stage JNAs. Endoscopic resection in experienced hands has the advantage of reducing hospital stays, decreasing intraoperative blood loss, and producing equal or reduced recurrence rates compared with open approaches.

Endoscopic-Assisted Approaches

Some studies have shown a benefit to combining endoscopic and open approaches in higher-stage JNAs.[8,33,44] Herman and colleagues[8] used a combined transfacial and endoscopic approach in 6 cases and reported that endoscopy led to the removal of JNA extensions that otherwise would have been left behind in traditional surgery. It was also implied that the use of endoscopy led to a decreased recurrence rate

---

Fig. 5. Endoscopic resection of a JNA. (*A*) Endoscopic view after an endoscopic medial maxillectomy performed to enhance intraoperative exposure. MMW, medial maxillary wall. (*B*) The intranasal portion of the JNA is debulked with the Coblator device (ArthroCare ENT, Sunnyvale, CA, USA). The coblator provides a near-bloodless field because it resects and coagulates the tumor at the same time. (*C*) The intranasal portion of the JNA has been removed, and the common sphenoid extension of the tumor is dissected away from the walls of the sphenoid sinus. SS, sphenoid sinus. (*D*) The tumor has been completely removed from the walls of the sphenoid sinus. The carotid prominences (CP) are noted for perspective. (*E*) The remaining portion of the JNA has been delivered to the nasopharynx and posterior nasal cavity with remaining attachments present at the sphenopalatine, clivus, and vidian canal. (*F*) The tumor has been completely extirpated by removing (and drilling) the clival attachments, sphenoid sinus floor, extensions into the pterygopalatine fossa (PPF), and vidian canal. (*G*) Postoperative endoscopic view at 9 months of clinical follow-up demonstrating no evidence of tumor recurrence. The pterygopalatine fossa and sphenopalatine area (*arrow*) are well healed, and the back wall of the sphenoid sinus is flush with the nasopharynx because of removal of a major portion of the clivus and sphenoid sinus floor. ET, eustachian tube.

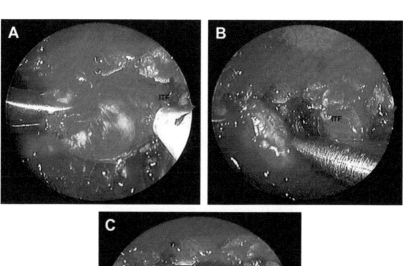

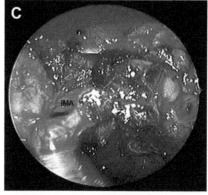

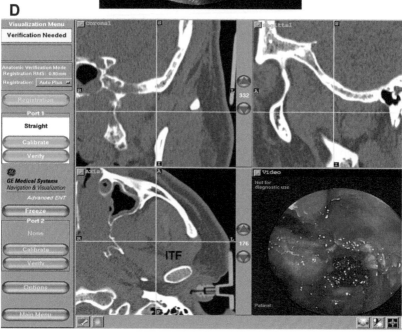

secondary to better visualization.[8] Combining endoscopy with traditional approaches usually decreases the extent of the open procedure and may eliminate the need for a second surgical approach to control larger tumors.[43] Hackman and colleagues[44] used a combined endoscopic and open (Caldwell-Luc) approach to allow for access to both central areas, such as the intranasal area, sphenoid, skull base, and cavernous sinus, and lateral extensions, such as the infratemporal fossa. The investigators felt that this combined approach gave wide access to the infratemporal skull base and masticator space. Three recurrences occurred in the combined group, but all were removed using a second endoscopic procedure.[44]

RECURRENCE: PREVENTION AND TREATMENT OF JNA

As reported previously, recurrence rates for JNAs range anywhere from 13% to 46% depending on the size, extent of tumor, and surgical approach.[35,43,46] Most tumors recur within 12 months of surgery.[10,33] Most investigators agree that recurrence rates correlate with the extent of the tumor, especially involvement of the skull base.[10,56] Herman and colleagues[8] reported that recurrence was most likely if the tumor involved the infratemporal fossa, sphenoid sinus, base of pterygoids and clivus, cavernous sinus, foramen lacerum, and anterior fossa. Most, if not all, recurrences can be attributed to incomplete tumor removal.[24,57] Howard and colleagues[35] was first to emphasize the importance of tumor extension into the sphenoid bone as an indicator of recurrence. On closer inspection, the investigators discovered interdigitations of angiofibroma in the cancellous bone of the sphenoid, which, if meticulously removed, significantly decreased their recurrence rates.[35] This finding has been duplicated in multiple studies and emphasizes the importance of extensive drilling of the basisphenoid if involved.[9,33,34,42] Because JNA is ultimately a benign tumor, many investigators support leaving the tumor behind if the remnant is located in an anatomically critical area (cavernous sinus, encasing the internal carotid artery).[8,33] Recurrence rates have some margin of error because many are usually tainted by growth of residual tumor thought to be a new recurrence. It can be difficult to know if a recurrence is actually new or just a growth of tumor left behind from a previous resection. In light of this, some advocate early postoperative imaging to identify residual disease for earlier treatment.[57]

Management of recurrence is controversial. Most agree that an easily accessible recurrence should be removed by a revision procedure (whether open or endoscopic).[2] In recurrent or residual intracranial disease, the decision must be made whether to subject the patient to a highly invasive procedure (craniotomy/endoscopy) with high morbidity or equally unappealing radiation therapy, which brings its own unique disadvantages to a young population. Both treatments have been used with success. Some advocate monitoring the recurrence/residual disease with imaging, and, if the tumor changes in size or becomes symptomatic, then treatment is initiated.[9] Another major factor is the possibility for JNAs to involute spontaneously

---

Fig. 6. (*A*) Because the extensions of angiofibromas do not invade the surrounding tissue, tumor may be dissected from difficult anatomic areas such as the infratemporal fossa (ITF). (*B*) This JNA was delivered from the ITF with retraction and blunt dissection using the team approach and underscores the improved access and operative efficiency using this technique in poorly accessible anatomic regions. (*C*) The tumor has been separated from the ITF, and the entrance of the embolized internal maxillary artery (IMA) into the tumor is visualized. (*D*) Triplanar CT image-guidance imaging and endoscopic view revealing the original location of the tumor in the infratemporal fossa. All attachments within the ITF and pterygopalatine fossa have been divided, and the JNA rests in the nasal cavity.

with time,[8,17,18,35] posing the question whether asymptomatic recurrences should be treated at all.

FOLLOW-UP IMAGING AFTER JNA RESECTION

Recommendations for follow-up after JNA resection vary widely depending on the institution. Most investigators use a combination of nasal endoscopy and MRI to detect recurrences, but timing and length of follow-up are inconsistent between investigators.[9,42] Mann and colleagues[28] advocate yearly MRIs and nasal endoscopy for at least 5 years postoperatively. Glad and colleagues[2] recommend a 6-month post-operative MRI and then a yearly follow-up afterward. However, evidence is shifting toward earlier postoperative imaging, within 1 month of surgery. The high incidence of residual disease (up to 40% in one study[57]) indicates that early detection of disease leads to better outcomes. Kania and colleagues[57] reported using contrast-enhanced CT scanning within 3 days of surgical excision to detect residual disease. They found that CT had a positive predictive value of 75% and specificity of 83% for detecting residual disease. The investigators contend that early detection of residual disease can usually be treated with minimally invasive surgery and thus decreases the need for repeat embolization or radiation therapy.[57] Because of this evidence, one investigator now performs an MRI scan on patients immediately after packing is removed. This MRI acts as a baseline to better differentiate postoperative recurrence versus scar tissue formation in later scans.[34] Chagnaud and colleagues[58] have suggested a protocol for surveillance of JNAs. If patients are asymptomatic and show no recurrence on imaging 3 to 4 months postoperatively, only a clinical examination is recommended. If clinical examination shows a possible recurrence either on endoscopy or imaging, further treatment should be performed with either radiation or surgery. If questionable recurrence is seen on 3- to 4-month postoperative imaging but endoscopic result is negative and the patient is asymptomatic, repeat imaging should be performed 3 to 6 months later. If the mass is of the same size or is smaller, repeat imaging should be performed in 6 months. If the mass enlarges, a second treatment of surgery or radiation is performed.[58]

SUMMARY

The optimal treatment of JNA must take into account multiple factors, including a young patient population, chance for spontaneous involution, surgical morbidity, radiation consequences, and risk of recurrence. The benign yet aggressive nature of the tumor causes a dilemma in management because the cure must not be worse than the disease. Endoscopic resection of JNAs may provide the ultimate solution to both predicaments. Endoscopic resection allows for complete resection of disease in many cases while providing the least morbidity. As endoscopic technology continues to develop, all tumors may eventually be treated exclusively with endoscopic techniques. It is only a matter of time before the endoscopic approach becomes the standard of care for most JNAs.

EBM Question	Author's reply
Is morbidity less with endoscopic resection (blood loss, cosmesis, CN injury, etc) compared to open surgery?	Evidence that endoscopic approaches have less morbidity than open approaches for the treatment of JNA exists with only 2 cohort studies directly comparing open with endoscopic techniques

REFERENCES

1. Chaveau UC. Histoire des Maladies du Pharynx. Arch Int Laryng 1906;21:889.
2. Glad H, Vainer B, Buchwald C, et al. Juvenile nasopharyngeal angiofibromas in Denmark 1981–2003: diagnosis, incidence, and treatment. Acta Otolaryngol 2007;127(3):292–9.
3. Beham A, Fletcher CD, Kainz J, et al. Nasopharyngeal angiofibroma: an immuno-histochemical study of 32 cases. Virchows Arch A Pathol Anat Histopathol 1993; 423(4):281–5.
4. Hwang HC, Mills SE, Patterson K, et al. Expression of androgen receptors in nasopharyngeal angiofibroma: an immunohistochemical study of 24 cases. Mod Pathol 1998;11(11):1122–6.
5. Schick B, Urbschat S. New aspects of pathogenesis of juvenile angiofibroma. Hosp Med 2004;65(5):269–73.
6. Lloyd G, Howard D, Lund VJ, et al. Imaging for juvenile angiofibroma. J Laryngol Otol 2000;114(9):727–30.
7. Lloyd G, Howard D, Phelps P, et al. Juvenile angiofibroma: the lessons of 20 years of modern imaging. J Laryngol Otol 1999;113(2):127–34.
8. Herman P, Lot G, Chapot R, et al. Long-term follow-up of juvenile nasopharyngeal angiofibromas: analysis of recurrences. Laryngoscope 1999;109(1):140–7.
9. Nicolai P, Berlucchi M, Tomenzoli D, et al. Endoscopic surgery for juvenile angio-fibroma: when and how. Laryngoscope 2003;113(5):775–82.
10. Bleier BS, Kennedy D, Palmer J, et al. Current management of juvenile naspoha-ryngeal angiofibroma: a tertiary center experience 1999–2007. Am J Rhinol Allergy 2009;23(3):328–30.
11. Andrews JC, Fisch U, Valavanis A, et al. The surgical management of extensive nasopharyngeal angiofibromas with the infratemporal fossa approach. Laryngo-scope 1989;99(4):429–37.
12. Chandler JR, Goulding R, Moskowitz L, et al. Nasopharyngeal angiofibromas: staging and management. Ann Otol Rhinol Laryngol 1984;93(4 Pt 1):322–9.
13. Radkowski D, McGill T, Healy GB, et al. Angiofibroma. Changes in staging and treatment. Arch Otolaryngol Head Neck Surg 1996;122(2):122–9.
14. Snyderman CH, Pant H, Carrau R, et al. A new endoscopic staging system for angiofibromas. Arch Otolaryngol Head Neck Surg 2010;136(6):588–94.
15. Labra A, Chavolla-Magaña R, Lopez-Ugalde A, et al. Flutamide as a preoperative treatment in juvenile angiofibroma (JA) with intracranial invasion: report of 7 cases. Otolaryngol Head Neck Surg 2004;130(4):466–9.
16. Jacobsson M, Petruson B, Ruth M, et al. Involution of juvenile nasopharyngeal an-giofibroma with intracranial extension. A case report with computed tomographic assessment. Arch Otolaryngol Head Neck Surg 1989;115(2):238–9.
17. Weprin LS, Siemers PT. Spontaneous regression of juvenile nasopharyngeal an-giofibroma. Arch Otolaryngol Head Neck Surg 1991;117(7):796–9.
18. Dohar JE, Duvall AJ 3rd. Spontaneous regression of juvenile nasopharyngeal an-giofibroma. Ann Otol Rhinol Laryngol 1992;101(6):469–71.
19. Tosun F, Onerci M, Durmaz A, et al. Spontaneous involution of nasopharyngeal angiofibroma. J Craniofac Surg 2008;19(6):1686–9.
20. Reddy KA, Mendenhall WM, Amdur RJ, et al. Long-term results of radiation ther-apy for juvenile nasopharyngeal angiofibroma. Am J Otolaryngol 2001;22(3): 172–5.
21. McAfee WJ, Morris CG, Amdur RJ, et al. Definitive radiotherapy for juvenile naso-pharyngeal angiofibroma. Am J Clin Oncol 2006;29(2):168–70.

22. Lee JT, Chen P, Safa A, et al. The role of radiation in the treatment of advanced juvenile angiofibroma. Laryngoscope 2002;112(7 Pt 1):1213–20.
23. Kuppersmith RB, The BS, Donovan DT, et al. The use of intensity modulated radiotherapy for the treatment of extensive and recurrent juvenile angiofibroma. Int J Pediatr Otorhinolaryngol 2000;52(3):261–8.
24. Marshall AH, Bradley PJ. Management dilemmas in the treatment and follow-up of advanced juvenile nasopharyngeal angiofibroma. ORL J Otorhinolaryngol Relat Spec 2006;68(5):273–8.
25. Wormald PJ, Van Hasselt A. Endoscopic removal of juvenile angiofibromas. Otolaryngol Head Neck Surg 2003;129(6):684–91.
26. Li JR, Qian J, Shan XZ, et al. Evaluation of the effectiveness of preoperative embolization in surgery for nasopharyngeal angiofibroma. Eur Arch Otorhinolaryngol 1998;255(8):430–2.
27. Herman B, Bublik M, Ruiz J, et al. Endoscopic embolization with onyx prior to resection of JNA: a new approach. Int J Pediatr Otorhinolaryngol 2011;75(1):53–6.
28. Mann WJ, Jecker P, Amedee RG. Juvenile angiofibromas: changing surgical concept over the last 20 years. Laryngoscope 2004;114(2):291–3.
29. Borghei P, Baradaranfar MH, Borghei SH, et al. Transnasal endoscopic resection of juvenile nasopharyngeal angiofibroma without preoperative embolization. Ear Nose Throat J 2006;85(11):740–3, 746.
30. Virgin FW, Bleier BS, Woodworth BA. Evolving materials and techniques for endoscopic sinus surgery. Otolaryngol Clin North Am 2010;43(3):653–72, xi.
31. Eloy JA, Walker TJ, Casiano RR, et al. Effect of coblation polypectomy on estimated blood loss in endoscopic sinus surgery. Am J Rhinol Allergy 2009;23(5): 535–9.
32. Ruiz J. Radiofrequency coblation symposium. Rhinology World Meeting. Philadelphia (PA), April 15–19, 2009.
33. Tyagi I, Syal R, Goyal A. Staging and surgical approaches in large juvenile angiofibroma—study of 95 cases. Int J Pediatr Otorhinolaryngol 2006;70(9):1619–27.
34. Nicolai P, Villaret AB, Farina D, et al. Endoscopic surgery for juvenile angiofibroma: a critical review of indications after 46 cases. Am J Rhinol Allergy 2010;24(2):e67–72.
35. Howard DJ, Lloyd G, Lund V. Recurrence and its avoidance in juvenile angiofibroma. Laryngoscope 2001;111(9):1509–11.
36. Hosseini SM, Borghei P, Borghei SH, et al. Angiofibroma: an outcome review of conventional surgical approaches. Eur Arch Otorhinolaryngol 2005;262(10):807–12.
37. Woodworth BA, Bhargave GA, Palmer JN, et al. Clinical outcomes of endoscopic and endoscopic-assisted resection of inverted papillomas: a 15-year experience. Am J Rhinol 2007;21(5):591–600.
38. Schlosser RJ, Woodworth BA, Gillespie MB, et al. Endoscopic resection of sinonasal hemangiomas and hemangiopericytomas. ORL J Otorhinolaryngol Relat Spec 2006;68(2):69–72.
39. Day TA, Beas RA, Schlosser RJ, et al. Management of paranasal sinus malignancy. Curr Treat Options Oncol 2005;6(1):3–18.
40. Lowlicht RA, Jassin B, Kim M, et al. Long-term effects of Le Fort I osteotomy for resection of juvenile nasopharyngeal angiofibroma on maxillary growth and dental sensation. Arch Otolaryngol Head Neck Surg 2002;128(8):923–7.
41. Andrade NA, Pinto JA, Nóbrega M, et al. Exclusively endoscopic surgery for juvenile nasopharyngeal angiofibroma. Otolaryngol Head Neck Surg 2007;137(3): 492–6.
42. Sciarretta V, Pasquini E, Farneti G, et al. Endoscopic sinus surgery for the treatment of vascular tumors. Am J Rhinol 2006;20(4):426–31.

43. Carrau RL, Snyderman CH, Kassam AB, et al. Endoscopic and endoscopic-assisted surgery for juvenile angiofibroma. Laryngoscope 2001;111(3):483–7.

44. Hackman T, Snyderman CH, Carrau R, et al. Juvenile nasopharyngeal angiofibroma: the expanded endonasal approach. Am J Rhinol Allergy 2009;23(1):95–9.

45. Kostrzewa JP, Sunde J, Riley KO, et al. Radiofrequency coblation decreases blood loss during endoscopic sinonasal and skull base tumor removal. ORL J Otorhinolaryngol Relat Spec 2010;72(1):38–43.

46. Danesi G, Panciera DT, Harvey R, et al. Juvenile nasopharyngeal angiofibroma: evaluation and surgical management of advanced disease. Otolaryngol Head Neck Surg 2008;138(5):581–6.

47. Woodworth BA, Palmer JN. Spontaneous cerebrospinal fluid leaks. Curr Opin Otolaryngol Head Neck Surg 2009;17(1):59–65.

48. Purkey MT, Woodworth BA, Hahn S, et al. Endoscopic repair of supraorbital ethmoid cerebrospinal fluid leaks. ORL J Otorhinolaryngol Relat Spec 2009; 71(2):93–8.

49. Banks CA, Palmer JN, Chiu AG, et al. Endoscopic closure of CSF rhinorrhea: 193 cases over 21 years. Otolaryngol Head Neck Surg 2009;140(6):826–33.

50. Woodworth BA, Prince A, Chiu AG, et al. Spontaneous CSF leaks: a paradigm for definitive repair and management of intracranial hypertension. Otolaryngol Head Neck Surg 2008;138(6):715–20.

51. Woodworth BA, Schlosser RJ. Repair of anterior skull base defects and CSF leaks. Op Tech Otolaryngol 2006;18:111–6.

52. Woodworth BA, Neal JG, Schlosser RJ. Sphenoid sinus cerebrospinal fluid leaks. Op Tech Otolaryngol 2006;17:37–42.

53. Woodworth BA, Schlosser RJ, Palmer JN. Endoscopic repair of frontal sinus cerebrospinal fluid leaks. J Laryngol Otol 2005;119(9):709–13.

54. Woodworth BA, Schlosser RJ, Faust RA, et al. Evolutions in the management of congenital intranasal skull base defects. Arch Otolaryngol Head Neck Surg 2004;130(11):1283–8.

55. Robinson S, Patel N, Wormald PJ. Endoscopic management of benign tumors extending into the infratemporal fossa: a two-surgeon transnasal approach. Laryngoscope 2005;115(10):1818–22.

56. Douglas R, Wormald PJ. Endoscopic surgery for juvenile nasopharyngeal angiofibroma: where are the limits? Curr Opin Otolaryngol Head Neck Surg 2006;14(1): 1–5.

57. Kania RE, Sauvaget E, Guichard J, et al. Early postoperative CT scanning for juvenile nasopharyngeal angiofibroma: detection of residual disease. AJNR Am J Neuroradiol 2005;26(1):82–8.

58. Chagnaud C, Petit P, Bartoli J, et al. Postoperative follow-up of juvenile nasopharyngeal angiofibromas: assessment by CT scan and MR imaging. Eur Radiol 1998;8(5):756–64.

Hypothalamic/ Pituitary Morbidity in Skull Base Pathology

Paul Lee, MBBS, FRACP, PhD[a,b], Ken K.Y. Ho, MD, FRACP[a,b,c],
Jerry R. Greenfield, MBBS, FRACP, PhD[d,e,f],*

KEYWORDS

- Hypothalamic dysfunction • Hypopituitarism • Skull base
- Craniopharyngioma

EBM Question	Level of Evidence	Grade of Recommendation
What is consequence of pituitary sacrifice in young patients (ie, craniopharyngioma)?	1b	A

The skull base is a complex anatomic region, which forms the floor of the cranial cavity, separating the brain from other facial structures. The ethmoid, sphenoid, occipital, paired frontal, and paired parietal bones divide up the skull base into the anterior, middle, and posterior cranial fossae. Each region contains vital neurovascular structures.

The middle fossa is of particular endocrine importance, as it nests the pituitary gland, or the hypophysis, which is a protrusion from the inferior surface of the hypothalamus. The hypothalamus is sometimes known as the "master clock" and the pituitary the "master gland." The hypothalamus regulates circadian rhythms by coordinating

[a] Department of Diabetes and Endocrinology, Princess Alexandra Hospital, 199 Ipswich Road, Woolloongabba, Brisbane, Queensland, Australia 4102
[b] School of Medicine, University of Queensland, 199 Ipswich Road, Woolloongabba, Brisbane, Queensland, Australia 4102
[c] Centres of Health Research, Princess Alexandra Hospital, 199 Ipswich Road, Woolloongabba, Brisbane, Queensland, Australia 4102
[d] Department of Endocrinology and Diabetes Centre, 390 Victoria Street, Darlinghurst, Sydney, New South Wales, Australia 2010
[e] Diabetes and Obesity Program, Garvan Institute of Medical Research, 384 Victoria Street, Darlinghurst, Sydney, New South Wales, Australia 2010
[f] Faculty of Medicine, University of New South Wales, Sydney, New South Wales, Australia 2052
* Corresponding author. Department of Endocrinology, Garvan Institute of Medical Research, 384 Victoria Street, Darlinghurst, Sydney, New South Wales, Australia 2010.
E-mail address: j.greenfield@garvan.org.au

Otolaryngol Clin N Am 44 (2011) 1005–1021
doi:10.1016/j.otc.2011.06.010
0030-6665/11/$ – see front matter © 2011 Elsevier Inc. All rights reserved.
oto.theclinics.com

endogenous biological oscillators with "time giver" signals, such as the light-dark cycle, to keep synchrony with the environment. Through the neurohypophyseal circulation, the hypothalamus communicates with the anterior pituitary gland, which secretes 6 hormones: growth hormone (GH), follicle-stimulating hormone (FSH), luteinizing hormone (LH), adrenocorticotropin (ACTH), thyroid-stimulating hormone (TSH), and prolactin. The posterior pituitary gland secretes anti-diuretic hormone (ADH) and oxytocin.

The hypothalamic-pituitary axis orchestrates a complex neuroendocrine circuitry with other endocrine glands, the principal ones being the thyroid, adrenals, and gonads, to regulate whole body homeostasis. These glands control essential body functions, including appetite, reproductive function, growth and development, energy metabolism, and water balance. Given their central and midline location, the hypothalamus and the pituitary gland are vulnerable to insults and damage by skull base pathologies and radiotherapy targeting the skull base. The most important consequences are hypothalamic dysfunction and hypopituitarism arising from hypothalamic and pituitary gland damage.

Hypothalamic dysfunction can cause disabling obesity, disorders of temperature regulation, or sleep disorders. Hypopituitarism refers to the deficiency of one or more pituitary hormones and results in a range of clinical syndromes with significant morbidity and mortality.[1,2] It is therefore important to diagnose and manage hypopituitarism early in order to improve both quality of life and survival.

In this review the epidemiology, pathophysiology, clinical presentation, investigation, management, and prognosis of hypopituitarism and hypothalamic dysfunction, arising from skull base pathologies and treatment of these conditions, are discussed. The clinical question "what is the consequence of pituitary hypofunction in young patients (ie, craniopharyngioma)?" is raised and answered.

HYPOPITUITARISM
Epidemiology

Limited information is available on the epidemiology of hypopituitarism in the general population. The prevalence of hypopituitarism was estimated to be 175, 290, and 450 cases per million in 3 cross-sectional surveys.[3–5] Even less information is available in patients with skull base pathologies, and most are limited to those who have received radiotherapy. Scattered case reports and series describe the development of hypopituitarism in patients following radiotherapy in the 1980s.[6–8] In these small series, the cumulative probability of varying degrees of hypopituitarism range from 60% to 100%. Pai and colleagues[9] reported a 10-year rate of hypopituitarism in 107 adults following radiotherapy to the skull base, the largest series to date, to be as high as 63%. Samaan and colleagues[10] studied 15 patients who had received radiotherapy for nasopharyngeal cancer, and found hypopituitarism to be present in 14 patients at 20 years' follow-up.

In the presence of hypopituitarism, mortality is increased. Data from 6 epidemiologic studies report increased mortality, with standardized mortality rates ranging from 1.2 to 2.2.[11,12] Excess mortality arises from cardiovascular and cerebrovascular diseases.[13] Patients with craniopharyngioma and/or patients treated with radiotherapy appear to be at higher risk.[1,2,14]

Pathophysiology

The most common cause of hypopituitarism in patients with skull base pathologies relates to local mass effect or treatment with radiotherapy.

Skull base mass lesions

Neoplasm is the most common skull base mass lesion. Compression of the pituitary stalk portal vessels by the neoplasm is the usual causative mechanism. The lesion can arise from the expanding neoplasm or secondary to an increase in intrasellar pressure.[15] Other mass lesions arise from developmental abnormalities such as craniopharyngiomas, Rathke cleft cysts, and arachnoid cysts. In addition to anterior pituitary hormone deficiencies, craniopharyngiomas can rarely cause diabetes insipidus, due to ADH deficiency.[16]

Craniopharyngiomas are the third most common intracranial tumor, and account for the majority of parapituitary tumors. There is a bimodal peak in incidence at age 5 to 14 years and again after the age of 50. The origin of their development is uncertain. There are frequently large cystic components and the tumors may be intrasellar, extrasellar, or both. Rathke cleft cysts are cystic sellar and suprasellar lesions lined by a single epithelial layer. Arachnoid cysts present at a later age, and are less common than both craniopharyngiomas and Rathke cleft cysts.

Derangement of central endocrine regulation also occurs with other parapituitary space-occupying lesions such as chondromas, suprasellar meningiomas, astrocytomas of the optic nerve, primary tumors of the third ventricle, and secondary metastases.

Radiotherapy

Radiation-induced damage to the hypothalamus and pituitary inevitably occurs when the hypothalamic-pituitary axis lies within the field of radiation. External cranial radiotherapy is commonly used in the treatment of nasopharyngeal carcinomas and parasellar tumors. Deficiency of one or more anterior pituitary hormones is almost invariable following radiotherapy. The most studied patient population has been patients with pituitary tumors treated with radiotherapy. Data are less comprehensive on patients with skull base neoplasms who receive radiotherapy, mainly because of the frequent omission of dynamic testing for GH and ACTH deficiency.

Unlike tumor cells, which are rapidly dividing and are therefore susceptible to nonrepairable "single-hit" radiation damage, the hypothalamic-pituitary axis is more vulnerable to cumulative sublethal radiation. The risk and severity of permanent hypopituitarism varies according to the total dose, the number of fractions, the duration of radiotherapy, and the length of follow-up. The relationship between these parameters and the risk of hypopituitarism was systematically evaluated in 107 adult patients who received radiotherapy (median dose 75 Gy) to the base of skull region for treatment of parasellar tumors.[9] In this study, patients were monitored for up to 10 years (median follow-up 5.5 years) for evidence of hypopituitarism. **Fig. 1** shows the Kaplan-Meier estimates of freedom from hypopituitarism following radiotherapy. Five-year actuarial rates of TSH, gonadotropin, and ACTH deficiency were 30%, 29%, and 19%, respectively, which rose to 63%, 36%, and 28% at 10 years. Among the patients who developed hypopituitarism, 47% had more than one axis involved. In a radiation dose analysis, the investigators identified a minimum target dose of 55 Gy as the threshold for pituitary damage, as no patients who received less than 55 Gy to the pituitary gland developed hormone deficiencies. Similar findings were reported in other smaller studies.[10,17]

Diabetes insipidus from ADH deficiency secondary to radiation is rare and has not been consistently reported. Hayashi and colleagues[18] reported a case series describing impaired ADH secretion in patients who received radiation doses as high as 140 to 180 Gy. Diabetes insipidus was transient, suggesting a much higher dose threshold for radiation-induced diabetes insipidus.

Collectively these studies highlight the importance of endocrine surveillance after radiotherapy to skull base regions, as only approximately 10% of patients were free

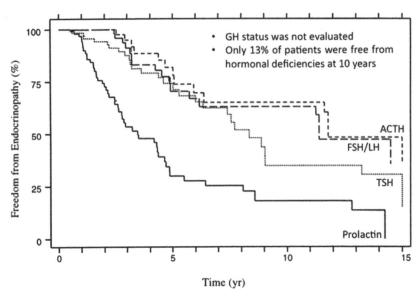

Fig. 1. Kaplan-Meier estimates of freedom from endocrinopathy following proton-photon beam radiotherapy. (*Adapted from* Pai HH, Thornton A, Katznelson L, et al. Hypothalamic/pituitary function following high-dose conformal radiotherapy to the base of skull: demonstration of a dose-effect relationship using dose-volume histogram analysis. Int J Radiat Oncol Biol Phys 2001;49(4):1079–92; with permission.)

from hypopituitarism at 10-year follow-up. However, there is one major limitation in these studies: the GH axis is frequently not evaluated. The somatotrophs are the most sensitive to radiation damage. Isolated GH deficiency occurs even after low radiation doses (<30 Gy) to the pituitary gland, and the frequency of GH deficiency rises to 50% to 100% at higher doses. In 2 studies comprising 43 patients with nasopharyngeal carcinomas followed for up to 17 years who underwent the insulin tolerance test (ITT), GH deficiency was diagnosed in up to 90% of patients.[6,8] The speed of onset of hormonal deficiency is also dependent on the radiation dose. GH deficiency occurs earlier with greater doses. For example, between 2 and 5 years after irradiation, all children receiving more than 30 Gy to the hypothalamic-pituitary axis developed subnormal GH responses to ITT, whereas more than one-third of children who received less than 30 Gy displayed a normal response.

One should be cautious in interpreting the impact of radiation-induced damage to the hypothalamic-pituitary axis on GH status. Depending on the tests used, discordant results may be seen in response to different GH-provocative agents. For example, a normal or mildly insufficient GH response during the combined GH-releasing hormone (GHRH) plus arginine stimulation test was seen in 50% of the patients classified as severely GH deficient using the ITT.[19,20] The choice and performance of different dynamic tests to evaluate GH sufficiency is discussed in greater detail in the section Investigations.

There is a theoretical advantage in using fractionated stereotactic conformal radiotherapy (SCRT) given the greater precision in irradiation localization, which may reduce radiation damage to normal structures in the brain. However, the incidence of hypopituitarism was not different between conventional radiotherapy and SCRT.[21,22] Close to a quarter of patients with previously normal pituitary function or partial hypopituitarism who received SCRT developed new hormonal deficit at a median follow-up of 32 months, and panhypopituitarism was seen in 18%.[22]

With the advances in the care in patients with skull base malignancies, survival of these patients has improved.[23] Therefore with increased survival, follow-up evaluation of patients irradiated for tumors of the skull base must focus equally on the possibility of tumor recurrence and the delayed effects of therapy, including the endocrine effects. Endocrine testing should be performed on a yearly basis for at least 10 years and again at 15 years.

Clinical Presentation

The presentation of hypopituitarism is affected by the degree, type, and rate of onset of the pituitary hormone deficiency. Symptoms and signs can be nonspecific and a high index of suspicion is required for diagnosis, which frequently necessitates measurement of basal hormone profile and sometimes dynamic endocrine testing. Radiation-induced hypothalamic-pituitary damage produces a characteristic evolution of pituitary failure of an initial loss of GH secretion, followed by gonadotropins, and finally by failure of ACTH and TSH secretion.

Hypopituitarism arising from radiation-induced damage to the hypothalamic-pituitary axis occurs over years, and the onset of symptoms is typically insidious. The nonspecific symptoms of lethargy, fatigue, low mood, and declining libido are common in cancer survivors and may be difficult to distinguish from symptoms of depression. In addition to cancer-induced cachexia, ACTH deficiency can cause anorexia and weight loss. **Table 1** summarizes the symptoms and signs of individual hormone deficiency. The features of isolated deficiencies of each axis are described below.

GH deficiency

There has been a recent reappraisal of the role of GH in adult health.[24] While the critical role of GH in stimulating childhood growth is well recognized, GH is the most abundant hormone in the adult pituitary gland and continues to be produced throughout adulthood. GH plays a general role in maintaining critical metabolic processes and the integrity of many tissues. GH deficiency is the earliest manifestation of many forms of hypopituitarism, such as radiation-induced hypothalamic-pituitary damage. However, it frequently remains undiagnosed because of the nonspecificity of the symptoms. Another common reason for overlooking the GH axis is the "myth" that GH replacement is contraindicated in patients with a history of malignancy. There is no convincing evidence for a causal link between GH treatment and tumor recurrence or the development of neoplasia.[25] The relationship between GH replacement and risk of malignancy recurrence is discussed in the section Management.

Before puberty, growth failure is the predominant feature of GH deficiency, which is distinct and rarely missed. Adult-onset GH deficiency is characterized by an impairment of psychological well-being and reduced quality of life. Common symptoms include fatigue, easy exhaustion, and lack of vitality. These patients display dry and atrophic skin, with a disproportionate increase in body fat and concomitant reduction of lean body mass, resulting in significant impairment of physical fitness and muscle strength.[24,26]

Gonadotropin deficiency

Gonadotropins are important for sexual development, function, and skeletal health. The presentation of hypogonadism is therefore different, depending on the age of individual patients.

In male patients the features are those of delayed puberty, characterized by small penis, small testes, and eunuchoid proportions (span exceeds height >5 cm). Men who have acquired gonadotropin deficiency postpubertally display reduced testicular

Table 1
Symptoms and signs of pituitary hormone deficiencies

Hormone	Symptom		Sign	
	Prepubertal	Postpubertal	Prepubertal	Postpubertal
Growth hormone	Growth failure	Loss of vitality, muscle weakness and fatigue, depression	Short stature	Increased fat mass, central adiposity, loss of lean mass, skin thinning and dryness
Gonadotropins	Delayed puberty	Loss of libido, sexual dysfunction, infertility	Delayed puberty	Loss of secondary sexual characteristics
TSH	Tiredness, cold intolerance, constipation, weight gain, depression, cognitive decline		Puffy face, periorbital edema, coarse skin, loss of eyebrows, delayed relaxation of tendon reflexes	
ACTH	*Chronic:* Tiredness, fatigue, weight loss, anorexia, myalgia, arthralgia *Acute:* Presentation can be catastrophic with circulatory shock		Hypotension (may be postural only)	
Prolactin	Failure to lactate			
ADH	Polydypsia, polyuria		Dehydration if intake does not match output	

volume and loss of secondary sexual characteristics, such as loss of facial and body hair and thinning of the skin. Other effects include gynecomastia, erectile dysfunction, and a decrease in skeletal muscle mass, bone mineral density, and general well-being. Azoospermia is found in all cases of hypogonadotropic hypogonadism.

In female patients, gonadotropin deficiency results in primary amenorrhea and absent breast development. In the adult woman, amenorrhea or oligomenorrhea, infertility, breast atrophy, vaginal dryness, and dyspareunia occur. As adrenal androgen production is regulated by ACTH action, a sign of ACTH deficiency is the loss of androgen-dependent pubic and axillary hair.

TSH deficiency

TSH deficiency occurs late in most pituitary disorders. Symptoms are generally milder than in primary hypothyroidism because of some residual TSH secretion. Hypothyroid symptoms include cold intolerance, weight gain, tiredness, and constipation, similar to those seen in primary hypothyroidism. Patients may appear edematous with a pulse at the lower end of the normal range. In severe hypothyroidism, bradycardia and myxedema can occur, although these are rare in patients with TSH deficiency.

ACTH deficiency

ACTH secretion is typically preserved until late in hypopituitarism. However, ACTH deficiency is life-threatening, and patients can present with profound shock if the onset is abrupt. Radiation-induced hypopituitarism usually causes chronic ACTH deficiency. The clinical presentation is characterized by slow and progressive symptoms of fatigue, anorexia, and weight loss. On examination, pallor is common with loss of secondary sexual hair, especially in females.

ADH deficiency

The classic features of diabetes insipidus from ADH deficiency are polydipsia and polyuria with nocturia. ADH deficiency can result in significant dehydration and hypovolemia if fluid intake is not increased to compensate for urinary loss.

Investigations

Diagnosis of hypopituitarism can be difficult, and frequently necessitates referral to an endocrine service with expertise in dynamic testing. Diagnosis in a patient with suspected hypopituitarism begins with history and clinical examination. A high index of suspicion is necessary for clinical diagnosis even among those with suggestive symptomatology, because of the nonspecific nature of symptoms.

In patients with skull base neoplasms who have received radiotherapy, the likelihood of hypothalamic-pituitary dysfunction is sufficiently high to warrant regular endocrine evaluation, even in the absence of typical symptoms. The risk of radiation-induced hypopituitarism is discussed in detail in the section Pathophysiology.

Evaluation of suspected hypopituitarism involves measurement of both baseline and stimulated hormone levels. Evaluation of baseline function includes prolactin, TSH, free thyroxine (T_4), cortisol, LH, FSH, and total testosterone in men and estradiol in women. Baseline blood testing reliably identifies hypogonadism, hypothyroidism, and severe hypoadrenalism due to pituitary insufficiency. **Table 2** summarizes the endocrine tests for each pituitary hormone deficiency.

In postmenopausal women with gonadotropin deficiency, gonadotropin levels are low or undetectable whereas in premenopausal women, low estradiol levels and low or normal gonadotropin levels, with a clinical presentation of amenorrhea or oligomenorrhea, are sufficient evidence of the diagnosis. In adult men, a similar picture of low testosterone levels and low or inappropriately normal gonadotropin levels is seen.

Table 2
Endocrine testing of pituitary hormone deficiencies

Hormone Deficiency	Screening Test	Confirmatory Test
Growth hormone	Serum IGF-1	Insulin tolerance test
Gonadotropins	Serum FSH, LH, estrogen (women), total testosterone (men)	Dynamic testing not necessary
TSH	Serum TSH, free T_4	
ACTH	Early-morning serum cortisol	Insulin-tolerance test
ADH	Paired serum and urine sodium, osmolality	Water-deprivation test

The biochemical picture of secondary hypothyroidism is similar to that seen in secondary hypogonadism. Free T_4 concentration is low, in association with a low or inappropriately normal serum TSH concentration.

Serum insulin-like growth factor 1 (IGF-1) concentration may be measured for evaluation of GH deficiency, but is only useful when age-adjusted normal ranges are used. While a low age-adjusted IGF-1 level is seen in adult GH deficiency, a normal concentration does not exclude the diagnosis. However, a subnormal IGF-1 level in an adult patient with coexisting pituitary hormone deficits is strongly suggestive of GH deficiency, particularly in the absence of conditions known to reduce IGF-1 levels such as malnutrition, liver disease, poorly controlled diabetes mellitus, and hypothyroidism. Patients with 3 or more pituitary hormone deficiencies and an IGF-1 level below the reference range have a greater than 97% chance of being GH deficient, and therefore do not require a GH stimulation test.[24]

Dynamic Testing

Provocative endocrine testing is indicated for those with suspected ACTH and GH deficiency, as basal hormonal profile does not distinguish those with mild to moderate deficiency from normal individuals. The ITT is the test of choice, as it evaluates for GH and ACTH deficiency concurrently. Following injection of a standard dose of intravenous insulin (0.1 unit/kg), GH and cortisol concentrations are serially measured. The ITT evaluates the response of the hypothalamic-pituitary-adrenal axis to the potent stressor of hypoglycemia, and is generally the gold standard in the confirmation of GH deficiency and secondary adrenal failure.

GH deficiency

Several provocative tests are available for the testing of GH deficiency. The ITT was recommended as the test of choice by the Growth Hormone Research Society.[24] Although the GHRH plus arginine test and the GHRH plus GH-releasing peptide test are valid alternatives to the ITT, both of these directly stimulate GH release from the pituitary gland and may miss GH deficiency due to hypothalamic disease. This finding is particularly relevant to radiation-induced hypothalamic-pituitary dysfunction, in which the ITT shows the greatest sensitivity and specificity within the first 5 years after irradiation, whereas false negatives may occur when GHRH-based tests are used.[19]

The ITT, which should be performed in experienced endocrine units under supervision, distinguishes GH deficiency from the reduced GH secretion that accompanies normal aging. Severe GH deficiency is defined by a peak GH response to hypoglycemia of less than 3 μg/L.[24]

ACTH deficiency

The highest plasma cortisol levels are found between 6:00 AM and 8:00 AM in normal individuals, and the lowest before midnight. If an early-morning cortisol level is less than 100 nmol/L, cortisol deficiency is highly likely, whereas a baseline level greater than 500 nmol/L indicates normality and thus dynamic testing may not be required.[27]

For patients with intermediate cortisol levels, ITT is indicated. On achievement of adequate hypoglycemia (<2.2 mmol/L), a peak cortisol response of between 500 and 600 nmol/L is generally accepted as adequate.[28]

The short Synacthen (tetracosactrin) test is not useful in the evaluation of pituitary reserve. An exogenous bolus of synthetic ACTH is a good test of adrenal reserve, but does not reliably detect ACTH deficiency, as in the case of radiation-induced hypopituitarism.

ADH deficiency

The diagnosis of ADH deficiency is suggested by the presence of polyuria (more than 40 mL/kg per 24 hours). To confirm the diagnosis, an 8-hour fluid-deprivation test is required, which should be performed under strict observation in an endocrine center, because of the risk of severe fluid and electrolyte depletion. In patients with ADH deficiency the urine fails to concentrate, resulting in a rapid increase in plasma osmolality.

Management

Endocrine replacement therapy to restore normal physiologic circulating hormone levels is the goal in hypopituitarism treatment. The aim is to mimic the normal hormonal milieu as far as possible, thus improving symptoms while avoiding overtreatment. The form and dose of hormone required depend on the physiologic need of each individual, which varies with age, gender, and health status. Endocrine replacement therapy for each anterior pituitary hormone is discussed in this section.

GH replacement

GH replacement stimulates protein synthesis, lipolysis, and fat oxidation, and reduces protein oxidation, which results in an increase in lean body mass and a decrease in fat mass.[29] Bone mineral density showed progressive increase up to 5%, with the level being twice as high in GH-treated subjects as in controls.[30,31] GH replacement also improved perceived health status, vitality, mood, and subjective well-being, which are frequent symptoms in patients with skull base malignancies.[29,32,33]

There has been concern that GH may increase the risk of tumor recurrence, given that GH promotes tissue growth. However, this concern is theoretical with no convincing supportive evidence. This risk of tumor progression or recurrence is unproven. In the Hypopituitary Control and Complications Study Italian Database, 90 patients with craniopharyngioma were treated with GH with no evidence of tumor regrowth.[34] There was no relationship between dose of GH and treatment modalities in more than 1000 patients with craniopharyngioma treated with GH for 10 years.[32] Chung and colleagues[35] prospectively followed 50 patients with a range of parasellar tumors in addition to craniopharyngioma, including germ cell tumor, arachnoid cyst, meningioma, glioma, and mesenchymal tumor, for 3 years, and GH replacement was abandoned in only 1 patient because of an apparent increase in tumor volume. In addition, overall cancer incidence rates in acromegalic patients were lower than those in the general population.[36] Collectively these data provide strong evidence against a causal association between GH replacement and an increased risk of malignancy.

GH replacement should be initiated and monitored by an endocrinologist with experience in the treatment of hypopituitarism. The starting dose of GH in young men and women is 0.2 and 0.3 mg/d, respectively, and in older individuals 0.1 mg/d.[24]

Subsequent monitoring of serum GH and IGF-1 levels guide dose escalation, which should be individualized and guided by clinical response.

The most common side effect of GH is fluid retention, which can manifest as edema, paresthesia, and carpal tunnel syndrome. The effects are usually mild and resolve either spontaneously or with dosage reduction.[37]

Sex-steroid replacement

Sex-steroid replacement maintains normal body composition, skeletal health, and sexual function in hypogonadal patients. It is therefore the most appropriate form of replacement therapy. Gonadotropin therapy is indicated only in patients planning pregnancy.

In women, estrogen is provided by many standard hormone-replacement therapies, together with progesterone, the latter in women with an intact uterus. A nonoral route (eg, transdermal, gel, or implant) is recommended because oral estrogen reduces hepatic IGF-1 production and worsens the metabolic impact of GH deficiency.[38]

For men various formulations of androgen replacement are available, and the choice of preparation depends on availability and patient preference. Recently, testosterone undecanoate, a long-acting intramuscular injection, has become available, providing stable serum testosterone levels for more than 3 months. This new preparation may therefore be more convenient than traditional short-acting intramuscular formulations and implants.

ACTH deficiency

Glucocorticoid requirement increases during acute illness. The goal of glucocorticoid replacement is to provide physiologic levels but to ensure sufficiency during times of acute illness. Different formulations are available, including hydrocortisone, cortisone acetate, prednisolone, and dexamethasone, with differing pharmacokinetics and pharmacodynamics. In general, the lowest replacement dose tolerated by the patient is preferred (equivalent to 10–20 mg cortisol per day). Doses should be divided to suit individual needs and overreplacement should be avoided, as it may worsen metabolic profile.[39]

It is of paramount importance that any patient identified as having ACTH deficiency should be educated about its clinical implications. An appropriate Medic-alert bracelet or necklace should be worn, and patients should be instructed to increase the replacement dose twofold to threefold in the case of an intercurrent illness or when undergoing surgery.

TSH deficiency

T_4-replacement therapy is the treatment of choice for TSH deficiency, and patients are treated in the same way as in primary hypothyroidism. The normal starting dose in a young patient without evidence of cardiac disease is 1.5 μg/kg/d. In a patient suspected to have hypopituitarism, T_4 therapy should be delayed until ACTH deficiency has been excluded or treated, as T_4 replacement may worsen cortisol deficiency if present. Measurement of TSH is unhelpful in the monitoring of T_4-replacement therapy in secondary hypothyroidism, and thyroxine dosage should be titrated according to serum free T_4 level.

ADH deficiency

Desmopressin is the drug of choice for the treatment of diabetes insipidus, and can be administered orally or intranasally. Desmopressin is commenced at a low dose and the dose increased according to clinical response. The aim is to control urine output, and the dose required can vary considerably between different patients. Serum sodium level should be monitored to prevent development of hyponatremia from overreplacement.

HYPOTHALAMIC DYSFUNCTION

The proximity of the hypothalamus to several skull base neoplasms, such as cranio-pharyngiomas, renders it vulnerable to damage by direct tumor infiltration, surgical insult, or radiation-induced dysfunction. The hypothalamus regulates important circadian and homeostatic body functions. It is responsible for integrating metabolic and environmental information regarding nutrient stores and circadian rhythmicity, with afferent sensory information about food availability and dark-light cycles.

Hypothalamic Obesity

Hypothalamic obesity is a rare syndrome in humans. When the ventromedial or para-ventricular region of the hypothalamus is damaged, hyperphagia develops and obesity follows, as seen in animal models.[40]

This syndrome can be caused by trauma, tumor, inflammatory disease, irradiation, or surgery in the posterior fossa. In a retrospective analysis of 52 patients, in which 22 were those with craniopharyngiomas, progressive weight gain was observed over a 5-year follow-up period since treatment.[41] The pathogenesis is unclear but has been attributed to hyperphagia, impaired sensitivity to satiety hormones, physical inactivity, and blunted thermogenesis.[42] These findings were supported by a series of 72 patients with hypothalamic obesity in which somnolence and thermodysregulation were seen in 55%.[43] Adjusted resting energy expenditure was lowered by 90 kcal per day, and physical activity reduced (**Fig. 2**) in 42 craniopharyngioma patients compared with matched controls.[44]

Disrupted Circadian Rhythms

Daytime hypersomnolence is a common presenting symptom of hypothalamic dysfunction. Disrupted sleep patterns were described in patients with craniopharyng-ioma, which stem from dysfunction of the hypothalamic circadian pacemaker in the suprachiasmatic nucleus.[45]

Clinical presentation is characterized by fatigue on a background of disordered sleep-wake architecture. Patients frequently have irregular bedtimes, unrestful sleep, frequent nighttime activities, and inappropriate daytime episodes of rest. This pattern may be further complicated by superimposed obstructive sleep apnea due to obesity. Among 79 patients with childhood craniopharyngioma, salivary concentration of melatonin, which is a marker of hypothalamic circadian function, correlated negatively with the patient's Epworth Sleepiness Scale score.[45] Mean 24-hour plasma melatonin levels were up to 25 times lower in craniopharyngioma survivors compared with controls.[46] These studies supported melatonin deficiency and irregular circadian function as mechanisms of hypersomnolence observed in hypothalamic dysfunction.

Management of Hypothalamic Dysfunction

Management of hypothalamic dysfunction is challenging. It necessitates a multidisciplinary team approach, involving the expertise of endocrinologists, dietitians, sleep physicians, and exercise physiologists. Given the profound impact on mood from disordered sleep and weight control, consultation from psychologists may be required.

A multifactorial approach involving a supervised program incorporating dietary and exercise intervention to achieve weight reduction, proper treatment of obstructive sleep apnea, and exposure to bright light on awakening to both improve energy level and consolidate sleep-wake rhythms, may be the most useful. Pharmacotherapy may be added as an adjunct to these behavioral interventions. Limited success has been

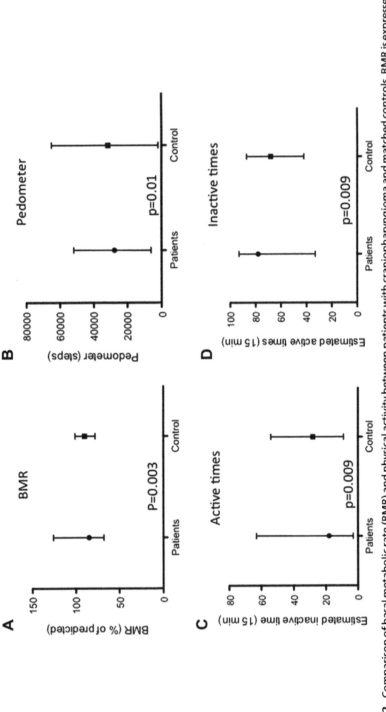

Fig. 2. Comparison of basal metabolic rate (BMR) and physical activity between patients with craniopharyngioma and matched controls. BMR is expressed as percentage of predicted (*A*). Physical activity is expressed as pedometer steps over a 3-day period (*B*), and estimated active time (*C*) and inactive time (*D*) in periods of 15-minute intervals. (*Adapted from* Holmer H, Pozarek G, Wirfalt E, et al. Reduced energy expenditure and impaired feeding-related signals but not high energy intake reinforces hypothalamic obesity in adults with childhood onset craniopharyngioma. J Clin Endocrinol Metab 2010;95(12):5395–402; with permission.)

reported with the use of stimulant and melatonin therapy to improve hypersomno-lence. Dexamphetamine, 5 mg twice daily, improved daytime wakefulness and stabi-lized weight in 10 of 12 patients in an observational series.[47] All 10 adult obese patients with childhood craniopharyngioma who received melatonin supplementation demon-strated reduction in daytime sleepiness.[48] These findings require confirmation in a larger number of patients before routine clinical use can be recommended.

CLINICAL QUESTION: WHAT IS THE CONSEQUENCE OF PITUITARY HYPOFUNCTION IN YOUNG PATIENTS (IE, CRANIOPHARYNGIOMA)?

Craniopharyngiomas are rare but aggressive tumors that arise from remnants of Rathke's pouch. These tumors comprise about 5% to 10% of all brain tumors in chil-dren. Patients are typically managed by a multidisciplinary team including surgeons and radiation oncologists, as treatment frequently entails neurosurgical resection fol-lowed by postoperative radiation therapy. A wide range of endocrine complications are observed in these patients following treatment, in addition to a close to twofold increase in mortality [Level 1b]. Hypopituitarism can arise in part from the original tumor but can be exacerbated by treatment, especially radiotherapy.

Hypopituitarism involving one or more anterior pituitary axes is present in the majority of young patients following treatment, and can be manifested by hypogonad-ism, hypothyroidism, adrenal insufficiency, or GH deficiency [Level 1b]. The conse-quences of each of these anterior pituitary hormonal deficiencies depend on the time of onset of hypopituitarism.

GH is the most commonly impaired pituitary axis in both childhood-onset and adult-onset hypopituitarism. Children who survive craniopharyngioma following surgery and radiotherapy are at significant risk of developing classic features of GH deficiency. Average final heights are expected to be 1 standard deviation below age, sex, and ethnically matched controls [Level 1b]. While somatic growth is no longer a concern for young patients who have developed GH deficiency after puberty, the main sequelae are decreased quality of life, adverse body-compositional changes charac-terized by an increase in fat mass and a decrease in lean mass and bone mineral density, higher risk of fracture, and worsened cardiovascular risk profile [Level 1b].

Gonadotropin deficiency is the second most common consequence in young patients who survive skull base malignancies. Manifestation is age-dependent and sex-dependent. Children may exhibit precocious puberty or delayed puberty. In post-pubertal patients, hypogonadotropic hypogonadism results in anovulatory cycles and hypoestrogenemia in women, and azospermia and hypoandrogenemia in men. Infer-tility is common. Chronic hypogonadism in both sexes results in weaning of secondary sexual characteristics, impaired sexual function, and osteoporosis [Level 1b].

TSH and ACTH secretion are least commonly impaired in radiation-induced hypo-pituitarism in patients with craniopharyngioma. These conditions are more likely consequences of direct surgical insult or if radiation doses are more than 55 Gy [Level 2b]. Untreated TSH deficiency leads to central hypothyroidism with fluid retention, cold intolerance, and lethargy. ACTH deficiency is usually of insidious onset with progressive anorexia, weight loss, low mood, and fatigue. These symptoms can be difficult to distinguish from the primary condition and may be mistaken as cancer cachexia [Level 1b].

ADH deficiency is rare following radiotherapy, but may arise from tumor infiltration or direct surgical insult [Level 4].

Hypothalamic dysfunction is also encountered in survivors of craniopharyngioma. These patients may develop morbid obesity, which is a consequence of hypothalamic

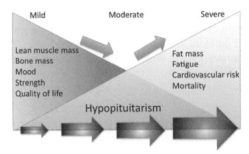

Fig. 3. Development of symptoms and body compositional abnormalities paralleling progressive loss of pituitary and hypothalamic functions over time.

damage causing disrupted or impaired sensitivity to feeding-related signals, and reduction in both metabolic rate and physical activity from hypersomnolence [Level 4].

SUMMARY

Hypothalamic-pituitary damage is common in patients with skull base pathologies. Hypothalamic dysfunction and hypopituitarism increase morbidity and mortality in affected patients (**Fig. 3**). Adequate and appropriate hormone replacement is mandatory in the management of hypopituitary patients. Management of hypothalamic obesity and hypersomnolence remains suboptimal, and further research is required to understand their pathogenesis and to guide treatment. The modern management of hypothalamic dysfunction and hypopituitarism should also focus on their prevention. By restricting surgery to experienced centers and replacing conventional radiotherapy for stereotactic surgery, the incidence of hypothalamic dysfunction and hypopituitarism will be reduced.

EBM Question	Author's reply
What is consequence of pituitary sacrifice in young patients (ie, craniopharyngioma)?	• There is a two-fold increase in mortality in those with pituitary dysfunction. • Hypopituitarism involving one or more anterior pituitary axes is present in the majority of young patients following treatment, and can be manifested by hypogonadism, hypothyroidism, adrenal insufficiency, or GH deficiency • Average final height are expected to be 1 standard deviation below age, sex and ethnically matched controls (GH deficiency) and increase in fat mass and a decrease in lean mass and bone mineral density, higher risk of fracture, and worsened cardiovascular risk profile(post somatic growth). • Chronic hypogonadism in both sexes results in weaning of secondary sexual characteristics, impaired sexual function, and osteoporosis • TSH and ACTH secretion are least commonly impaired post radiation • ADH deficiency is rare post radiation or from direct tumour involvement (Level 4) • Morbid obesity can occur post therapy from impaired sensitivity to feeding-related signals, and reduction in both metabolic rate and physical activity from hypersomnolence (Level 4)

REFERENCES

1. Sherlock M, Ayuk J, Tomlinson JW, et al. Mortality in patients with pituitary disease. Endocr Rev 2010;31(3):301–42.
2. Tomlinson JW, Holden N, Hills RK, et al. Association between premature mortality and hypopituitarism. West Midlands Prospective Hypopituitary Study Group. Lancet 2001;357(9254):425–31.
3. Regal M, Paramo C, Sierra SM, et al. Prevalence and incidence of hypopituitarism in an adult Caucasian population in northwestern Spain. Clin Endocrinol (Oxf) 2001; 55(6):735–40.
4. Nilsson B, Gustavasson-Kadaka E, Bengtsson BA, et al. Pituitary adenomas in Sweden between 1958 and 1991: incidence, survival, and mortality. J Clin Endocrinol Metab 2000;85(4):1420–5.
5. Stochholm K, Gravholt CH, Laursen T, et al. Incidence of GH deficiency—a nationwide study. Eur J Endocrinol 2006;155(1):61–71.
6. Lam KS, Ho JH, Lee AW, et al. Symptomatic hypothalamic-pituitary dysfunction in nasopharyngeal carcinoma patients following radiation therapy: a retrospective study. Int J Radiat Oncol Biol Phys 1987;13(9):1343–50.
7. Lam KS, Tse VK, Wang C, et al. Early effects of cranial irradiation on hypothalamic-pituitary function. J Clin Endocrinol Metab 1987;64(3):418–24.
8. Lam KS, Wang C, Yeung RT, et al. Hypothalamic hypopituitarism following cranial irradiation for nasopharyngeal carcinoma. Clin Endocrinol (Oxf) 1986; 24(6):643–51.
9. Pai HH, Thornton A, Katznelson L, et al. Hypothalamic/pituitary function following high-dose conformal radiotherapy to the base of skull: demonstration of a dose-effect relationship using dose-volume histogram analysis. Int J Radiat Oncol Biol Phys 2001;49(4):1079–92.
10. Samaan NA, Bakdash MM, Caderao JB, et al. Hypopituitarism after external irradiation. Evidence for both hypothalamic and pituitary origin. Ann Intern Med 1975;83(6):771–7.
11. Bates AS, Van't Hoff W, Jones PJ, et al. The effect of hypopituitarism on life expectancy. J Clin Endocrinol Metab 1996;81(3):1169–72.
12. Svensson J, Bengtsson BA, Rosen T, et al. Malignant disease and cardiovascular morbidity in hypopituitary adults with or without growth hormone replacement therapy. J Clin Endocrinol Metab 2004;89(7):3306–12.
13. Brada M, Ashley S, Ford D, et al. Cerebrovascular mortality in patients with pituitary adenoma. Clin Endocrinol (Oxf) 2002;57(6):713–7.
14. Karavitaki N, Wass JA. Craniopharyngiomas. Endocrinol Metab Clin North Am 2008;37(1):173–93, ix-x.
15. Arafah BM, Prunty D, Ybarra J, et al. The dominant role of increased intrasellar pressure in the pathogenesis of hypopituitarism, hyperprolactinemia, and headaches in patients with pituitary adenomas. J Clin Endocrinol Metab 2000;85(5): 1789–93.
16. Crowley R, Hamnvik O, O'Sullivan E, et al. Morbidity and mortality in craniopharyngioma patients after surgery. Clin Endocrinol (Oxf) 2010;73:516–21.
17. Jensen RL, Jensen PR, Shrieve AF, et al. Overall and progression-free survival and visual and endocrine outcomes for patients with parasellar lesions treated with intensity-modulated stereotactic radiosurgery. J Neurooncol 2010;98(2): 221–31.
18. Hayashi M, Chernov MF, Taira T, et al. Outcome after pituitary radiosurgery for thalamic pain syndrome. Int J Radiat Oncol Biol Phys 2007;69(3):852–7.

19. Darzy KH, Aimaretti G, Wieringa G, et al. The usefulness of the combined growth hormone (GH)-releasing hormone and arginine stimulation test in the diagnosis of radiation-induced GH deficiency is dependent on the post-irradiation time interval. J Clin Endocrinol Metab 2003;88(1):95–102.

20. Darzy KH. Radiation-induced hypopituitarism after cancer therapy: who, how and when to test. Nat Clin Pract Endocrinol Metab 2009;5(2):88–99.

21. Hoybye C, Grenback E, Rahn T, et al. Adrenocorticotropic hormone-producing pituitary tumors: 12- to 22-year follow-up after treatment with stereotactic radio-surgery. Neurosurgery 2001;49(2):284–91 [discussion: 291–2].

22. Minniti G, Traish D, Ashley S, et al. Fractionated stereotactic conformal radio-therapy for secreting and nonsecreting pituitary adenomas. Clin Endocrinol (Oxf) 2006;64(5):542–8.

23. Zada G, Laws ER. Surgical management of craniopharyngiomas in the pediatric population. Horm Res Paediatr 2010;74(1):62–6.

24. Ho KK. Consensus guidelines for the diagnosis and treatment of adults with GH deficiency II: a statement of the GH Research Society in association with the European Society for Pediatric Endocrinology, Lawson Wilkins Society, European Society of Endocrinology, Japan Endocrine Society, and Endocrine Society of Australia. Eur J Endocrinol 2007;157(6):695–700.

25. Allen DB. Safety of human growth hormone therapy: current topics. J Pediatr 1996;128(5 Pt 2):S8–13.

26. Ho KK. Diagnosis of adult GH deficiency. Lancet 2000;356(9236):1125–6.

27. Le Roux CW, Meeran K, Alaghband-Zadeh J. Is a 0900-h serum cortisol useful prior to a short synacthen test in outpatient assessment? Ann Clin Biochem 2002;39(Pt 2):148–50.

28. Nieman LK. Dynamic evaluation of adrenal hypofunction. J Endocrinol Invest 2003;26(Suppl 7):74–82.

29. Bengtsson BA, Eden S, Lonn L, et al. Treatment of adults with growth hormone (GH) deficiency with recombinant human GH. J Clin Endocrinol Metab 1993; 76(2):309–17.

30. Johannsson G, Rosen T, Bosaeus I, et al. Two years of growth hormone (GH) treatment increases bone mineral content and density in hypopituitary patients with adult-onset GH deficiency. J Clin Endocrinol Metab 1996;81(8):2865–73.

31. Shalet SM, Shavrikova E, Cromer M, et al. Effect of growth hormone (GH) treat-ment on bone in postpubertal GH-deficient patients: a 2-year randomized, controlled, dose-ranging study. J Clin Endocrinol Metab 2003;88(9):4124–9.

32. Darendeliler F, Karagiannis G, Wilton P, et al. Recurrence of brain tumours in patients treated with growth hormone: analysis of KIGS (Pfizer International Growth Database). Acta Paediatr 2006;95(10):1284–90.

33. Maiter D, Abs R, Johannsson G, et al. Baseline characteristics and response to GH replacement of hypopituitary patients previously irradiated for pituitary adenoma or craniopharyngioma: data from the Pfizer International Metabolic Database. Eur J Endocrinol 2006;155(2):253–60.

34. Cannavo S, Marini F, Trimarchi F. Patients with craniopharyngiomas: therapeutical difficulties with growth hormone. J Endocrinol Invest 2008;31(Suppl 9):56–60.

35. Chung TT, Drake WM, Evanson J, et al. Tumour surveillance imaging in patients with extrapituitary tumours receiving growth hormone replacement. Clin Endocri-nol (Oxf) 2005;63(3):274–9.

36. Orme SM, McNally RJ, Cartwright RA, et al. Mortality and cancer incidence in acromegaly: a retrospective cohort study. United Kingdom Acromegaly Study Group. J Clin Endocrinol Metab 1998;83(8):2730–4.

37. de Boer H, Blok GJ, Popp-Snijders C, et al. Monitoring of growth hormone replacement therapy in adults, based on measurement of serum markers. J Clin Endocrinol Metab 1996;81(4):1371–7.
38. Meinhardt UJ, Ho KK. Regulation of growth hormone action by gonadal steroids. Endocrinol Metab Clin North Am 2007;36(1):57–73.
39. Filipsson H, Monson JP, Koltowska-Haggstrom M, et al. The impact of glucocorticoid replacement regimens on metabolic outcome and comorbidity in hypopituitary patients. J Clin Endocrinol Metab 2006;91(10):3954–61.
40. Stefater MA, Seeley RJ. Central nervous system nutrient signaling: the regulation of energy balance and the future of dietary therapies. Annu Rev Nutr 2010;30:219–35.
41. Daousi C, Dunn AJ, Foy PM, et al. Endocrine and neuroanatomic features associated with weight gain and obesity in adult patients with hypothalamic damage. Am J Med 2005;118(1):45–50.
42. O'Gorman CS, Simoneau-Roy J, Pencharz Mb P, et al. Delayed ghrelin suppression following oral glucose tolerance test in children and adolescents with hypothalamic injury secondary to craniopharyngioma compared with obese controls. Int J Pediatr Obes 2010. [Epub ahead of print].
43. Bray GA, Gallagher TF Jr. Manifestations of hypothalamic obesity in man: a comprehensive investigation of eight patients and a review of the literature. Medicine (Baltimore) 1975;54(4):301–30.
44. Holmer H, Pozarek G, Wirfalt E, et al. Reduced energy expenditure and impaired feeding-related signals but not high energy intake reinforces hypothalamic obesity in adults with childhood onset craniopharyngioma. J Clin Endocrinol Metab 2010;95:5395–402.
45. Muller HL, Handwerker G, Wollny B, et al. Melatonin secretion and increased daytime sleepiness in childhood craniopharyngioma patients. J Clin Endocrinol Metab 2002;87(8):3993–6.
46. Lipton J, Megerian JT, Kothare SV, et al. Melatonin deficiency and disrupted circadian rhythms in pediatric survivors of craniopharyngioma. Neurology 2009;73(4):323–5.
47. Ismail D, O'Connell MA, Zacharin MR. Dexamphetamine use for management of obesity and hypersomnolence following hypothalamic injury. J Pediatr Endocrinol Metab 2006;19(2):129–34.
48. Muller HL, Handwerker G, Gebhardt U, et al. Melatonin treatment in obese patients with childhood craniopharyngioma and increased daytime sleepiness. Cancer Causes Control 2006;17(4):583–9.

References

Index

Note: Page numbers of article titles are in **boldface** type.

A

Adenomas, pituitary. See *Pituitary adenomas*.
Adrenocorticotropin deficiency, in hypopituitarism, 1011, 1013
Angiofibroma, nasopharyngeal juvenile. See *Nasopharyngeal angiofibroma(s), juvenile*.
Anti-diuretic hormone deficiency, in hypopituitarism, 1011, 1013

B

B_2-Transferrin, in detection of cerebrospinal fluid leak, 861
Beta-trace protein, in detection of cerebrospinal fluid leak, 861

C

Cerebrospinal fluid, functions of, 858
   normal physiology of, 846
Cerebrospinal fluid leaks, cerebrospinal fluid diversion in, 864
   classification of, 858
   clinical questions concerning, 868–869
   conservative management of, 863–864
   detection of, 860–861
   epidemiology of, 868–860
   following functional endoscopic sinus surgery, 859, 866
   following nonsurgical trauma, 869–870
   following surgical trauma, 870
   from benign intracranial hypertension, 859
   from tumor obstruction, 859
   identification of, 861
   in ethmoid/cribriform fracture, 869
   localization of, 861–863
   presenting signs of, 860–861
   reduction of cerebrospinal fluid pressure and, 850
   spontaneous, evaluation of, clinical presentation and, 846–847, 848
      in meningoceles, 849
      outcomes, intracranial pressure and, 850–852, 853
      pathophysiology of, 848–850
   surgical management of, 864–868
      endoscopic endonasal approach for, 865–866
      extracranial approach for, 865
      in surgical defects, 866–868
      transcranial approach for, 864
      transnasal approach for, 863
   traumatic, **857–873**
      meningitis following, 868–869

Otolaryngol Clin N Am 44 (2011) 1023–1028
doi:10.1016/S0030-6665(11)00120-4
oto.theclinics.com
0030-6665/11/$ – see front matter © 2011 Elsevier Inc. All rights reserved.

Moving?

Make sure your subscription moves with you!

To notify us of your new address, find your **Clinics Account Number** (located on your mailing label above your name), and contact customer service at:

Email: journalscustomerservice-usa@elsevier.com

800-654-2452 (subscribers in the U.S. & Canada)
314-447-8871 (subscribers outside of the U.S. & Canada)

Fax number: 314-447-8029

Elsevier Health Sciences Division
Subscription Customer Service
3251 Riverport Lane
Maryland Heights, MO 63043

*To ensure uninterrupted delivery of your subscription, please notify us at least 4 weeks in advance of move.

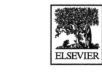

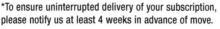

Printed and bound by CPI Group (UK) Ltd, Croydon, CR0 4YY

03/10/2024

01040457-0020